Surgical pathology revision

Second edition

This very popular revision guide, originally published in its first edition as *General Pathology Vivas*, is packed with useful information in A–Z format, covering the essentials of pathology for examination candidates. This accessible and informative text will help to dispel some of the anxiety facing those studying for their viva or oral examinations. It has been written by a pathologist with many years of experience teaching pathology. This new edition includes many updated and new entries to provide even broader coverage of the key topics and concepts that are an essential prerequisite to understanding basic surgical pathology. This concise account is aimed at undergraduate medical candidates and for the oral parts of the MRCS, MRCP and FRCOG examinations. It will also serve as a valuable aide memoire for the junior surgeon or doctor at all levels of experience, especially those training junior staff themselves.

D0300539

Surgical pathology revision

Second edition

DAVID LOWE
Harley Street, London

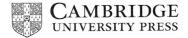

CAMBRIDGE
UNIVERSITY PRESS

CAMBRIDGE UNIVERSITY PRESS
Cambridge, New York, Melbourne, Madrid, Cape Town, Singapore, São Paulo, Delhi

Cambridge University Press
The Edinburgh Building, Cambridge CB2 8RU, UK
Published in the United States of America by Cambridge University Press, New York

www.cambridge.org
Information on this title: www.cambridge.org/9780521683586

First published by Greenwich Medical Media Ltd 2001
Reprinted 2003, 2004, 2005
This edition published 2006
Reprinted 2007
Reprinted with corrections 2009

Printed in the United Kingdom at the University Press, Cambridge

A catalogue record for this publication is available from the British Library

ISBN 978-0-521-68358-6 paperback

Medical disclaimer
Every effort has been made in preparing this publication to provide accurate and
up-to-date information which is in accord with accepted standards and practice
at the time of publication. Although case histories are drawn from actual cases,
every effort has been made to disguise the identities of the individuals involved.
Nevertheless, the authors, editors and publishers can make no warranties that
the information contained herein is totally free from error, not least because
clinical standards are constantly changing through research and regulation. The
authors, editors and publishers therefore disclaim all liability for direct or
consequential damages resulting from the use of material contained in this
publication. Readers are strongly advised to pay careful attention to information
provided by the manufacturer of any drugs or equipment that they plan to use.

Preface

Examination candidates appear for viva examinations in varying degrees of terror. In many cases the candidates obviously know the facts but have difficulty recalling them – they have no pegs to hang their ideas on. In some cases, they can recall but launch into their responses with little thought of classification or prioritisation. Some candidates have never sat a viva examination before, and it shows.

This book is intended for all of these candidates when they sit an examination that is on, or involves, surgical pathology. The construction of the entries follow that used by most examining bodies in their viva examinations. The topic is introduced by a relatively broad question to settle the candidate down, then more searching questions are asked to sound the depths of their knowledge. Questions on classification are popular as they show whether the candidate is able to think clearly and logically, and give relatively common examples early and keep the rarer ones until later. Another popular form is to make a question justify itself: 'Why should a surgeon know something about gout?' neatly establishes that a surgical candidate should be able to answer the question even though he or she had thought that gout was a medical topic.

Some of the entries ask questions and give responses that would almost certainly be considered too difficult for most junior qualifying examinations. These have been included for those candidates who like to leave a little leeway between just passing the examination and passing comfortably. Conversely, though the entries cover most of the likely topics asked on general pathology, the examiners may always come up with something new relevant to their own specialism. "Unseen" questions can still be tackled along the standard lines of the entries here: classify, give examples with the commonest first, discuss the complications.

The entries as arranged alphabetically so that topics can be found easily. As a consequence, the topics are usefully randomised, as the questions in a typical viva would be. I hope that the book will make a nerve-wracking experience more bearable.

David Lowe
London, 2006

■ Abscess and pus

What is an abscess?

An abscess is a localised tissue collection of pus. If pus forms
in the pleural space or peritoneum it may be loculated and so
considered to be an abscess (such as an appendix abscess or
subdiaphragmatic abscess) or lie free and be an empyema or
purulent generalised peritonitis.

What tissue is the wall of an abscess characteristically composed of?

Granulation tissue. This used to be called the "*pyogenic
membrane*", but it is not a true membrane and is not itself
pyogenic.

What is pus?

Pus is the product of acute inflammation composed of
cellular and fluid, exudative phases. When the cause of pus
formation is infective, the *solid* phase consists of:

- Live and dead polymorphs
- Live and dead macrophages
- Live and dead bacteria or other causative agent
- Dead human epithelial and connective tissue cells from the
  tissues involved in the acute inflammation
- A fibrin meshwork on which macrophages function much
  better

The *fluid* phase of pus is an exudate, which consists of water that permits migration of inflammatory cells and carries:

- Immunoglobulins for opsonisation
- Complement components for anaphylaxis, chemotaxis, opsonisation and membrane damage
- Clotting cascade factors which result in the fibrin meshwork above
- Inflammatory mediators other than the above such as arachidonic acid, kinins, cytokines

When the abscess is a sterile abscess micro-organisms are absent. Causes of sterile abscess include:

- Intramuscular injection of irritant pharmaceutical agents such as paraldehyde (historical only: no longer used therapeutically)
- Sterilisation by antimicrobials of a septic abscess

What is the natural history of an abscess?

To discharge itself through a line of least resistance.

What does the osmotic pressure of a solution depend on?

On the number of molecules present.

In pus, the number of these molecules increases constantly. Why?

Because of enzymes released from polymorphs and macrophages which split long-chain molecules such as proteins into smaller fragments. Then these fragments are further split, so the osmotic pressure increases until there is discharge of the pus into a hollow viscus, along fascial lines, into the peritoneal or other potential cavity, or out through the skin or mucous membranes.

■ Acromegaly

What is the definition of acromegaly?

The effects of excess growth hormone in an adult body (i.e. in a patient beyond the age at which bone and other normal growth has ceased).

What are the causes of acromegaly?

- Human growth hormone (hGH) secreted from an adenoma of the anterior pituitary (from chromophobe or acidophil cells called *somatotrophs*)
- Very rarely ectopic secretion of hGH from carcinoma of the pancreas, lung or small intestine

What surgically important diseases are associated with acromegaly?

- Osteoporosis and fractures
- Orthodontic procedures because of abnormality of bite
- Increased incidence of neoplastic large bowel polyps and adenocarcinoma of large bowel:
  - mediated by the actions of insulin-like growth factors from the liver
- Increased incidence of gall stones and gall bladder disease
- Increased incidence of hernia
- Increased incidence of the complications of diabetes mellitus
- Complications of reconstructive and related surgery

■ Actinomycosis

Why should a surgeon know about actinomycosis?
- Affects the neck (most commonly) and also the thorax, appendix, peritoneal cavity and central nervous system (CNS)
- Causes a local swelling with abscess formation, local fibrosis, and sinuses draining the area
- Can mimic a malignant neoplasm leading to overtreatment with consequent morbidity and mortality
- Relatively rare, usually responds to penicillin though a prolonged period of treatment is necessary
- Commoner in men than women, for no apparent reason
- Rare in children and people over 60 years

What pathogens characteristically cause actinomycosis?
- *Actinomyces israelii* is the commonest. The others (*Actinomyces naeslundii*, *Actinomyces odontolyticus*, *Actinomyces meyeri*) are rare
  - Gram-positive, anaerobic, filamentous bacteria
  - Commensal in the oral cavity, alimentary tract and female genital system
  - No risk of person-to-person spread of actinomycosis

What factors predispose to actimomycosis?
- Pathogenic only when there is tissue damage
  - Oral, facial and cervical involvement is characteristically only after dental operations, direct trauma or local sepsis from other organisms
  - Pulmonary involvement usually follows aspiration of oral, pharyngeal or upper gastrointestinal fluids

- Alimentary involvement is usually associated with breakdown of the mucosal barrier by appendicitis, diverticulitis, operative surgery and other trauma, or occasionally foreign bodies
- In the female genital system, infection has been linked with use of an intrauterine device, whether for contraception or hormone-replacement therapy

What is its characteristic course?
- Indolent
- Progressively forms fibrous tissue, multiple abscess, sinuses and fistulae
- Associated with pain, weight loss, fever, palpable mass, obstruction
- Often confused with malignancy

How may the diagnosis be suspected at the time of surgery?
- Yellow "sulphur granules"
  - Seen in pus in less than half of cases
  - Not pathognomonic
- Most cases are diagnosed post-operatively
- The organism takes a long time to grow: the patient's history and clinical findings should be discussed with a microbiologist

How may the diagnosis be made pre-operatively?
By a high index of suspicion and fine needle aspirate.

There are no serological or skin-sensitivity tests that will help in diagnosis. The main problem is to distinguish actinomyces infection from nocardia infection.

■ Adrenocortical insufficiency and Addison's disease

What is Addison's disease?

Adrenocortical insufficiency as a result of extensive bilateral destruction of the layers of the adrenal cortices. Thomas Addison (1793–1860) of Guy's Hospital, London described the disease in 1849 and 1855. His patients had bilateral adrenal tuberculosis.

How many anatomical layers does the adrenal have?

Three:

- Zona glomerulosa which secretes aldosterone
- Zona fasciculata–reticularis i.e. one zona which secretes cortisol and sex hormones
- Medulla

What are the causes of adrenocortical insufficiency?

- Infective with bilateral severe involvement of the adrenal glands
  - Tuberculosis
  - Fungal infections such as coccidioidomycosis, blastomycosis
- Infective with adrenal destruction as a secondary feature
  - Waterhouse–Friderichsen syndrome from meningococcal septicaemia
- Deposition
  - Extensive bilateral involvement by metastatic carcinoma

- Haemochromatosis
- Amyloidosis
- Autoimmune adrenalitis
- Iatrogenic
  - Bilateral adrenalectomy (as part of the treatment of breast carcinoma or Cushing's syndrome caused by ectopic adrenocorticotropic hormone (ACTH) secretion from an unidentified primary site) with inadequate replacement
  - Adrenolytic drugs such as *o-p*-dichlorodiphenyl-dichloroethane (*o-p*-DDD) and ketoconazole without replacement
  - Metyropone treatment without replacement
  - Sudden withdrawal of long-term steroid therapy

What are the clinical features of Addison's disease?
- Weight loss
- Ill-defined malaise
- Skin pigmentation especially in palmar creases, scars, genitalia and nipples, and on light exposed areas. The pigmentation occurs because of the reactive increase in pro-opiomelanocortin (POMC), from the anterior pituitary with increase in MSH (melanocyte-stimulating hormone) and ACTH as a consequence

What are the biochemical changes in the serum of patients with Addison's disease?
- Hyponatraemia
- Hyperkalaemia
- Increased serum ACTH
- Decreased serum aldosterone, cortisol

■ AIDS and neoplasia

What neoplasms characteristically occur in patients with AIDS?

- Lymphoma, of which the type is:
  - Commonly a B-cell non-Hodgkin's lymphoma (NHL)
  - Less commonly a T-cell NHL
  - Occasionally, an unusual aggressive form of Hodgkin's lymphoma that arises in sites that would be unusual for Hodgkin's disease in patients who do not have AIDS
- Skin neoplasms
  - Squamous cell papilloma, often with atypical appearances
  - Squamous cell carcinoma, especially of the skin of the anus and vulva
- Cervical neoplasms
  - Squamous cell carcinoma of cervix
- Laryngeal neoplasms
  - Squamous cell carcinoma of larynx

Toxoplasmosis can mimic a solitary brain neoplasm such as astrocytoma or a cerebral cyst. Kaposi's sarcoma, classically involving the skin, anus, large bowel and elsewhere is now considered to be a reactive process caused by human herpes simplex virus type 8.

What type of virus is HIV?

An RNA retrovirus that requires reverse transcriptase. It has core protein and RNA surrounded by a glycoprotein envelope and infects cells via CD4 receptors.

How may HIV be associated with a surgical "acute abdomen"?

- Bacterial enteritis
- Haemorrhage or other complications from Kaposi's sarcoma of gastrointestinal tract (GIT)
- Cytomegalovirus (CMV) infection of colon with megacolon
- Involvement of the GIT by lymphoma, classically NHL
- Infection of the GIT by mycobacteria, especially atypical mycobacteria, such as *Mycobacterium avium intracellulare* (MAI)
- By chance, such as appendicitis and diverticulitis

■ Alcohol-related disease

What are the physiological and pathological effects of ethyl alcohol on the body?

It affects principally the CNS, the stomach and pancreas, the larynx and the liver.

What are the hepatic changes as a consequence of excessive alcohol consumption?

- Fatty change, once considered innocuous and now considered to be damaging
- Alcoholic hepatitis with liver cell damage
- Cirrhosis, classically micronodular unless the person then gives up drinking, when it becomes mixed and then macronodular
- Hepatocellular carcinoma

How is alcohol metabolised by the liver?

- Microsomal ethanol oxidising system enzymes principally
- Alcohol dehydrogenase
- Catalase reaction

All of these reactions metabolise ethyl alcohol to acetic acid.

What CNS effects of alcohol would come to surgical notice?

- Head injury with the risk of intracranial haemorrhage
- Road traffic accidents, other physical trauma
- Cerebellar degeneration
- Korsakov's psychosis

- Incidentally in patients with surgically important disease when a patient has memory loss, confabulation, depression, abuse of other substances

What gastric and pancreatic diseases are associated with excessive alcohol consumption?
- Gastritis
- Gastric erosions and ulcers
- Acute pancreatitis
- Chronic pancreatitis
- Carcinoma of the pancreas

What laryngeal diseases are associated with consumption of undiluted spirits?
- Laryngeal inflammation
- Squamous cell carcinoma of the larynx

What other conditions are associated with excess alcohol ingestion?
- Squamous cell carcinomas of the pharynx and oesophagus, especially from drinking undiluted spirits
- Macrocytosis on blood film
- Tuberculosis and other infections of debilitated patients
- Impotence

■ Alternatives to blood transfusion

To reduce the risks of blood transfusion reactions, what alternatives are there to transfusion of whole blood?

- Consider the level at which blood products are required
  - 8 g/dl is considered an adequate haemoglobin concentration for most patients
  - For platelets, 10×10^9/l is considered adequate
  - Use fresh frozen plasma only to treat proven coagulopathies
- Avoid blood loss in the first instance
  - Diathermy, maintenance of normothermia
  - Fibrin sealant or glue: a mixture of fibrinogen, factor XIII, thrombin, aprotinin and calcium chloride
  - Anti-fibrinolytic agents: tranexamic acid, aprotinin
- Use haematinics and erythropoietin to correct anaemia preoperatively
  - For erythropoietin to be effective, iron and folate supplements should be given as well
- Use plasma expanders
  - Crystalloids, colloids
- Use autologous transfusion

What is meant by acute normovolaemic haemodilution?

A type of autologous transfusion

- Blood is taken from the patient during the induction of anaesthesia

- Colloid or crystalloid are given as concurrent replacement
- The patient's red cell mass is diluted; the low haematocrit reduces the number of red cells lost in the surgical procedure
- Blood taken at the start is replaced at the end of the procedure when surgical haemostasis has been achieved

What other techniques of autologous transfusion can be used?

- Pre-operative autologous deposit of whole blood
  - Four weeks before elective surgery, blood is taken from patients who have normal haemoglobin levels
  - A maximum of four units can be taken at weekly intervals
  - The procedure should not be undertaken unless there is a definite, guaranteed-as-far-as-possible date for the surgery
  - Supplementary iron and folate may be necessary
  - In practice the wastage rate of saved blood is high (in the USA, about half)
- Intra-operative red cell salvage
  - Shed blood from the operative field is collected and re-transfused
  - All systems filter the blood before return
    - Some send it straight back
    - Some wash the blood to remove haemolysed cells, free haemoglobin and other debris
    - Side effects include air embolism, coagulation abnormalities and disseminated intravascular coagulopathy

◼ Amoebiasis

What are the names of the organisms commonly known as amoebae?

Entamoeba histolytica and *Entamoeba coli.*

Which is the pathological one?

Principally *Entamoeba histolytica. Entamoeba coli* is a commensal or transitory organism in people in some parts of the world.

How may the entamoebae be distinguished histologically?

Entamoeba histolytica is tissue invasive and ingests red cells, which can be identified within the organism on microscopy. *Entamoeba coli* does not invade tissues or ingest red cells.

What diseases are caused by amoebae?

These include:

- Alimentary and related organs
  - Amoebic dysentery
  - Large bowel inflammatory polyps
  - Liver abscess (containing brown "anchovy sauce" pus)
- Skin involvement
  - Anal and vulval ulceration
- CNS involvement
  - Brain abscess
  - Meningoencephalitis (caused by *Naegleria fowleri*, another type of amoeba)

What are the further complications of amoeba infection?

- Cutaneous amoebiasis (vulval, anal, elsewhere)
- Peritonitis
  - *Amoeboma*: a tumour-like mass composed of inflammatory tissue containing very numerous amoebae which classically occurs in the large bowel
- Misdiagnosis as:
  - Squamous cell carcinoma of vulva or anus
  - A neoplastic polyp of large bowel

■ Amyloidosis I: classification

What is amyloid? Where does the term derive from?

First described by Rokitansky in 1842, though Virchow gave it the name "starch-like".

Amyloid is a family of unusual proteins, all of which have a characteristic β-pleated sheet structure which is unusual in biology. Most mammalian systems have no enzymes that will denature this family of compounds. On staining with Congo red, all members of the family have apple-green birefringence (dichroic birefringence) under polarised light.

The name amyloid derives from the blue-violet colour that tissues with amyloid deposits take on when exposed to iodine and a dilute acid. Iodine alone stains amyloid mahogany brown; addition of dilute sulphuric, hydrochloric or other acid turns the colour blue-violet.

How is amyloid classified?

By the protein involved, principally into AL and AA types of generalised amyloidosis and locally as Aβ in CNS, calcitonin in medullary carcinoma of thyroid and idiopathic localised deposits.

- AL amyloid, also known as amyloid of immune origin and used to be called *primary amyloid*
  - The soluble precursors are immunoglobulin light chains, especially λ chains from myeloma
  - Full immunoglobulins (usually IgG and IgA) may also be secreted
  - Heavy chains are sometimes found

- AA amyloid, also known as amyloid secondary to chronic inflammation and used to be called *secondary amyloid*
  - Results from macrophage secretion of interleukins, especially IL1 and IL6, that stimulate hepatocytes to secrete serum amyloid protein A (SAA) which is a normal acute phase protein. It is also the soluble amyloid precursor
- Aβ amyloid is found adjacent to the neurofibrillary tangles in Alzheimer's disease

What are the complications of amyloid?

AL amyloid affects:

- *Heart*: restrictive heart muscle disease (no longer called a *cardiomyopathy*)
- *Nerves*: generalised neuropathy or relatively selective involvement resulting in impotence, hypotension, and abnormalities of sweating
- *Skin*: microscopical deposits in dermal arteriolar walls, between collagen bundles in the dermis, and deeper as a cause of carpal–tunnel syndrome

AA amyloid affects:

- *Kidney*: renal arteries and arterioles, glomeruli, renal tubules causing nephrotic syndrome and chronic renal failure
- *Liver*: in the space of Diss; impairment of hepatic function is rare
- *Spleen*: around penicillary arteries ("sago spleen") or diffusely; impairment of function is rare

In many patients there is no good distinction of these separate patterns. The terminology of primary and secondary amyloidosis has been dropped as there is a great overlap of complications between the two main types.

■ Amyloidosis II: diagnosis and complications

From where would you take a biopsy to diagnose generalised amyloidosis?

The rectal submucosa – the biopsy must be deep enough to include muscular walled vessels which are found only in the submucosa and not the mucosa. A deep biopsy from the oral cavity would be informative but much more painful.

Give examples of diseases that result in AA amyloid.

- Chronic infections: tuberculosis, syphilis, leprosy, bronchiectasis, chronic osteomyelitis
- Chronic inflammatory diseases that may be infective; Whipple's disease, Reiter's syndrome
- Other chronic inflammatory diseases:
  - Rheumatoid arthritis – the commonest cause of amyloidosis in the UK
  - Ulcerative colitis and Crohn's disease
  - Longstanding paraplegia with immobility
- Neoplasms
  - Hodgkin's disease
  - Renal parenchymal cell carcinoma

What congenital causes of amyloidosis are there?

- The commonest is familial Mediterranean fever, which is an autosomal-recessive condition
- Portuguese-type amyloidosis

Can amyloid be found as localised deposits without generalised involvement?

- Endocrine gland amyloid in
  - *Medullary carcinoma of thyroid*: the amyloid is composed of calcitonin
  - *The pancreatic islets in diabetes mellitus*: the amyloid is composed of calcitonin gene-related peptide and other peptides
- Urinary tract amyloid
  - Solitary deposits of amyloid can occur anywhere in the urinary tract
- Laryngeal amyloid
  - Solitary deposits of amyloid can occur anywhere in the region of the larynx

Why is amyloid not metabolised by the body?

The human body has no enzymes that metabolise β-pleated sheets. For the same reason, silk in ligatures is very poorly metabolised and so persists for a long time.

■ Anaerobic organisms

What is the commonest commensal organism in the large bowel?

Bacteroides species outnumber *Escherichia coli.*

How can anaerobic organisms be classified?

Into obligate anaerobes, which can grow only in the absence of oxygen, and facultative anaerobes which can grow in the presence or absence of oxygen (a genus such has *Clostridium* has species of both types).

Give some examples of anaerobes.

- Gram-positive bacilli
  - *Clostridium* spp.
- Gram-negative bacilli
  - *Bacteroides* spp.
  - *Fusobacterium* spp.

What diseases are caused by anaerobes?

- Gas gangrene
- Pseudomembranous colitis
- Tetanus
- Botulism
- Abdominal sepsis, usually in cooperation with coliforms
- Sepsis in the gynaecological tract
- Dental and oropharyngeal disease

How would you strongly suspect that a wound was contaminated by anaerobic organisms?

From the smell, which is characteristic and dreadful.

■ Aneurysms

What is the definition of an aneurysm?
An abnormal localised dilatation of a blood vessel including arteries, arterioles, veins and the heart (aneurysmal dilatations of lymphatics can occur but are very rare).

How are aneurysms classified?
- True or false:
  - Whether the full thickness consisting of all three layers of the vessel wall is represented, a true aneurysm, or only a part, a false aneurysm (vascular surgeons use the terms differently from pathologists)
- Congenital or acquired:
  - A berry aneurysm of the anterior communicating branch of the circle of Willis is caused by a congenital deficiency though is manifest only in adult life. Hypertension is not a contributory cause, though these patients may develop hypertension due to associated polycystic disease
- By shape:
  - Saccular if only part of the circumference is involved
  - Fusiform if the entire circumference is involved
  - Dissecting when the arterial media is deficient as in syphilis, Erdheim's cystic medial necrosis and Marfan's syndrome (the aorta is an elastic artery, not a muscular artery)
- By cause:
  - *Atheroma*: descending aorta below the renal arteries
  - *Syphilis*: dissecting aneurysm of the ascending and arch of the aorta as a result of thrombosis of the vasa vasorum

secondary to inflammation in these vessels caused by the treponemes

- *Traumatic*: subclavian aneurysm related to a cervical rib, arteriovenous aneurysm from a penetrating injury, dissecting aneurysm from deceleration trauma
- *Inflammatory other than the above*: polyarteritis nodosa (PAN), aortitis in ankylosing spondylitis
- *Ischaemic*: ventricular aneurysm after myocardial infarction
- *Congenital*: berry aneurysm, cirsoid venous aneurysm on the scalp which is an aneurysmal hamartoma
- *Mycotic*: muscular arteries from low-grade bacterial infection (only very rarely fungal infection, as the name suggests)
- *Hypertension*: microaneurysms (Charcot–Bouchard aneurysms) in the brain
- *Iatrogenic*: arteriovenous (AV) aneurysm after dialysis shunt

What are the complications of aneurysm?

These include:

- Thrombosis
- Embolism
- Pressure effects
  - Pressure from an aneurysm of the arch of the aorta on the oesophagus, recurrent laryngeal nerve, vertebral column and sternum
  - Venous obstruction from pressure on the inferior vena cava (IVC)
- Haemorrhage from rupture, or dissection and rupture
- Ischaemia

▪ Apoptosis

What does apoptosis mean?

Apoptosis is the degradation of a cell to balance mitosis in regulating the size and function of the tissue, or to eliminate damaged cells with abnormal DNA. This process is energy dependent and does not stimulate an inflammatory response. Apoptosis may be physiological or as the result of a pathological process.

In apoptosis there is no:

- Failure of normal control mechanisms, as apoptosis is a normal event
- Passive change: apoptosis requires energy and specific protein synthesis
- Rupture of plasma membranes
- Inflammatory reaction

How is apoptosis considered to be a physiological process in the body?

- Embryologically there is loss of tissues between digits at certain times in development
- Physiological degeneration of the thymus occurs by apoptosis
- Cells are removed from the bowel mucosa normally when they are recognised as degenerate
- In the endometrial cycle, apoptosis removes cells when there is withdrawal of hormonal support
- After the menopause and after other withdrawal of trophic stimuli apoptosis occurs in the target organs such as the uterus, prostate and breast

How is apoptosis considered to be involved in the pathological processes of the body?

- Duct obstruction: apoptosis occurs in the affected glands such as the pancreas and parotid gland (but not the testis after vasectomy).
- Damage to cells from viruses, irradiation, drugs, other physical agents and T-lymphocytes as in graft rejection.
- As a reaction to abnormalities that occur in the normal cell cycle that require that the cell should be eliminated.
- In tumours, especially Burkitt's lymphoma, neuroblastoma and other rapidly proliferating but not rapidly growing neoplasms, the rate of apoptosis may be high and almost equal to the rate of tumour cell division.

How is apoptosis regulated?

- By gene products that protect against apoptosis (such as *bcl-2* and interleukins)
- By gene products that promote apoptosis (such as p53, *myc*)

■ Appendicitis

Most cases of appendicitis are idiopathic but occasionally a cause is found. How do you classify the causes of appendicitis?

As causes in the lumen, in the wall and outside the wall of the appendix.

- In the lumen causing predominantly mucosal appendicitis:
  - Worms:
    - *Enterobius vermicularis* (debated – usually incidental but occasionally causally related)
    - *Strongyloides stercoralis*
    - *Ascaris lumbricoides*
  - Tropical parasites such as oesophagostomiasis
  - Foreign material
- In the wall causing predominantly transmural appendicitis:
  - Infection:
    - Viral infections (especially adenovirus and CMV)
    - Bacterial infections such as tuberculosis, yersinia infection, actinomycosis
    - Amoebiasis
    - Schistosomes and other tropical parasites
  - Inflammation other than primarily infective:
    - Ulcerative colitis
    - Crohn's disease
    - Pseudomembranous colitis

- Ischaemia:
  - Ischaemic colitis
  - Congenital stricture
  - Iatrogenic causes
- Vascular abnormalities:
  - Angioma
  - Angiodysplasia
  - Vasculitides such as SLE (systemic lupus erythematosus) and PAN
  - Other congenital abnormalities
- Hamartoma:
  - Obstruction by a Peutz–Jeghers' polyp
- Neoplasia:
  - Pseudomyxoma of the appendix
    - Associated with mucocele of the appendix
    - Associated with mucinous and other neoplasms of the ovaries
  - Carcinoma of the appendix
  - Carcinoid of the appendix
  - Carcinoma of the caecum with obstruction
  - Lymphoma
- Outside the wall causing predominantly serosal appendicitis:
  - Salpingitis, oophoritis
  - Endometriosis
  - Diverticular disease
  - Generalised acute peritonitis
    - Uraemia
    - Gynaecological complications

- Autoimmune diseases such as rheumatoid arthritis
  and PAN
- Others:
  - Septicaemia
  - (Familial tendency)

■ Asbestos

What diseases are caused by asbestos?
- Carcinoma of bronchus, usually squamous cell carcinoma
- Malignant mesothelioma of pleura, pericardium and peritoneum
- Asbestosis – a fibrosing lung disease
- Chronic bronchitis as from any dust-related disease
- Misdiagnosis of pleural fibrous plaques as malignancy with consequent morbidity

In which occupations are people exposed to asbestos?
- Shipworkers
- Laggers, industrial plumbers
- Builders
- Workers in old institutions such as hospitals that have insulation that was installed over 50 years ago

What types of asbestos cause disease?
There are over 50 types of asbestos. Only three are of importance in disease:
- Chrysotile
  - *White asbestos*: accounts for 90% of asbestos used in industry
  - Woolly long fibres
  - Classified differently from the other two asbestoses in current use as a serpentine mineral rather than an amphibole

- Crocidolite
  - Blue asbestos
  - Straight short fibres
  - Associated with malignancy and fibrosis
  - Classified as an amphibole mineral
- Amosite
  - Brown asbestos
  - Straight long brittle fibres
  - Associated with fibrosis
  - Classified as an amphibole mineral

Why is crocidolite or blue asbestos worse than the other types?

Crocidolite fibres are short and straight, and so penetrates more deeply into the lungs, pericardium and peritoneum than the longer fibres of the other types of asbestos.

■ Ascites

What is ascites?
An abnormal amount of free fluid in the peritoneal cavity.

What are the causes of ascites?
- Causes of a transudate which accumulates as ascites:
  - Hydrostatic changes
    - Cirrhosis (the fluid escapes through the capsule of the liver)
    - Right-sided cardiac failure
    - Budd–Chiari syndrome
    - Obstruction of the thoracic duct (chylous ascites)
  - Plasma oncotic changes
    - Liver failure with hypoproteinaemia
    - Protein losing enteropathy
    - Starvation
    - Nephritic and nephrotic syndromes
  - Metabolic changes
    - Secondary hyperaldosteronism (though not primary, Conn's syndrome)
    - Hypothyroidism
- Causes of an exudate which accumulates as ascites:
  - Inflammatory causes resulting in protein leakage
    - Peritonitis
    - Peritoneal infiltration by carcinoma
    - Severe uraemia
    - Pancreatitis

- Iatrogenic
  - Operative abdominal surgery, which often results in some excess free fluid
  - Chronic airways limitation

What investigations can be carried out on ascitic fluid to ascertain the cause of the ascites?

- Microbiology:
  - Microscopy for bacteria, white cells, red cells
  - Culture and sensitivity (including for TB)
- Cytology microscopy for:
  - Involvement by metastatic or primary carcinoma
  - Involvement by lymphoma such as NHL
- Cytogenetics where appropriate
- Biochemistry for:
  - Amylase if pancreatitis is suspected
  - Protein content

■ Atheroma I: tissue changes

How is arteriosclerosis classified?

Into:

- Atheroma (a much better term than atherosclerosis, which is an oxymoron)
- Arteriolosclerosis, such as caused by diabetes mellitus and hypertension
- Monkeberg's median sclerosis of medium-sized arteries, classically in the pelvis

What is atheroma?

Atherosclerosis is a disease of elastic and medium-sized muscular arteries down to 1 mm in diameter. It characteristically comprises:

- Endothelial changes with interactions among platelets, white cells and myofibroblasts
- Inflammation of the affected artery wall
- Build-up of lipids, cholesterol, calcium and cellular debris in the artery's intima
- Plaque formation
- Increasing luminal obstruction
- Abnormal blood flow
- Ischaemia in severe cases

What causes the tissue changes in atheroma?

Essentially unknown. Likely to be a cascading response to endothelial cell injury with free radical formation as a result of:

- Low-density lipoprotein (LDL) cholesterol

- Overwhelms the antioxidant properties of the endothelial cells
- Impairs the capacity to dilate and contract
- Toxins, including cigarette smoke
- Hyperglycaemia
- Hyperhomocystinaemia

Macrophage contribution:
- Circulating monocytes infiltrate the intima and become macrophages
- Macrophages ingest LDL cholesterol to form characteristic foam cells with intracellular lipid
- Secretion of cytokines and other substances from the activated macrophages further injure the endothelium

Increased tendency for thrombus formation:
- Increased platelet adhesion, decreased plasminogen activator

Haemodynamic factors:
- Shear stresses from blood flow affect gene expression in endothelial cells
- Plaques occur where blood flow changes in velocity and direction

What are the classic lesions that affect the artery?
- The fatty streak as above
- The fibrous plaque
  - Progressive lipid accumulation
  - The migration and proliferation of myofibroblasts
  - Mitogens from platelets, macrophages and affected endothelial cells

- Smooth muscle cells form the connective tissue in the fibrous cap
- Below this there are foam cells, extracellular lipid and cellular debris
- Growth of the plaque results in:
    - Increasing luminal narrowing
    - Further abnormalities of blood flow
    - Ischaemia of the organ supplied
    - The advanced or complicated lesion
    - Rupture of the fibrous cap
    - Weakening by T-lymphocytes secreting interferon gamma
    - Macrophages produce metalloproteinases that degrade collagen
    - Thrombus formation with partial or complete occlusion
    - Progression of the atheroma by organisation of the thrombus and incorporation within the plaque

A | **Atheroma I: tissue changes**

■ Atheroma II: epidemiology and complications

What are the age and sex differences in atheroma?
- Atheroma is commoner in men
  - Lack of protection by oestrogen and progesterone
- The incidence of coronary heart disease in women parallels that in men but 10 years later
- Most patients with idiopathic atheroma develop symptoms and signs after the age of 50 years

What are the causes and associations of atheroma formation?
- Hyperlipidaemia
- Hypertension
  - A risk factor for the development of atheroma and stroke
  - The mechanism is unknown
- Diabetes mellitus
  - Commonly associated with hypertension, coagulopathies and abnormalities of endothelial cells
- Cigarette smoking
  - Endothelial dysfunction
  - Hypercoagulable state
- C-reactive protein (CRP) concentration in the plasma
  - CRP reflects systemic inflammation which may play a role in the pathogenesis and progression of atheroma
  - Risk factor modification: aspirin and human menopausal gonadotropin co-enzyme A (HMG-CoA) reductase inhibitors may reduce plaque inflammation

- Homocysteine concentration in the plasma
  - Patients with hyperhomocystinaemia have widespread atheroma at an early age
- Fibrinogen concentration in the plasma
  - Fibrinogen may be increased by smoking and with age and diet and so may be a covariable
  - Independently, raised concentrations of fibrinogen are a strong predictor of cardiovascular damage
  - This association seems as strong as that between hypercholesterolaemia and coronary artery disease
- Lipoprotein A concentration in the plasma
  - Raised concentrations of lipoprotein A have been found to have an association with coronary artery disease

What are the complications of atheroma?

The serious complications include:

- Ischaemia from gradual obstruction
- Occlusion of a vessel (characteristically a coronary artery) because of:
  - Progressive accumulation of lipid in the atheromatous plaque
  - Rupture of a plaque causing instant thrombosis
  - Haemorrhage into a plaque causing instant thrombosis
  - Lipid embolus from a plaque causing thrombosis distal to it
- Embolus of thrombus formed over an atheromatous plaque
- Aneurysm formation

■ Atrophy, aplasia, agenesis

What do the terms agenesis, aplasia, hypoplasia and atrophy mean?

- *Agenesis*: the complete failure of an organ or tissue to develop in any way.
- *Aplasia and hypoplasia*: the failure of an organ or tissue to attain its proper size, state or function, though there is an attempt at this. In aplasia, there is recognisable tissue that has failed to develop; in hypoplasia, development has proceeded further but has not reached normal maturity. *Atresia* is a form of aplasia: it is the failure of the development of a lumen in a normally hollow structure such as the choanae, bile ducts or intestine.
- *Atrophy*: the degeneration of an organ or tissue from its normal, fully formed state to a state in which there is reduction in the normal cell size, cell number, or both.

Give examples of aplasia and agenesis.

- Agenesis in branchial pouch development can result in failure of parathyroid glands and thymus to develop.
- Aplasia of a lung in a child, with emphysema as a compensatory mechanism.

Classify the causes of atrophy.

- Physiological:
  - Fetal and early childhood
    - Notochord
    - Thyroglossal duct

- Branchial clefts
- Ductus arteriosus
- Umbilical vessels
- Fetal layer of the adrenal cortex
  - Later childhood
    - Thymus
  - Adulthood
    - Uterus and vagina after the menopause
    - Breasts after the menopause
    - Lymphoid tissue is gradually replaced by adipose tissue
- Pathological:
  - Generalised
    - Starvation
  - Specific
    - Osteoporosis
    - Ischaemia
    - Pressure effects
    - Disuse: immobilisation, CNS defects, obstruction
    - Neuropathic after lower motor neurone lesions
    - Idiopathic: testicular atrophy, Alzheimer's disease

■ Autoimmune diseases

How are autoimmune diseases classified?
Organ specific and non-organ specific.

Give some examples of autoimmune disease that are not organ specific, with the relevant antigens.
- *Rheumatoid arthritis*: IgG
- *Systemic lupus erythematosus*: DNA and several other cell components
- *Discoid lupus erythematosus*: nuclear antigens other than DNA
- *Primary biliary cirrhosis*: mitochondria
- *Chronic active hepatitis*: smooth muscle

Give some examples of autoimmune disease that are organ specific, with the relevant antigens.
- *Hashimoto's thyroiditis*: thyroid antigens (multiple)
- *Graves' disease*: thyroid-stimulating hormone (TSH) receptors
- *Pernicious anaemia*: intrinsic factor in parietal cells
- *Autoimmune adrenalitis*: components of adrenal cortical cells
- *Idiopathic thrombocytopaenic purpura*: platelets
- *Myasthenia gravis*: acetylcholine receptor antibodies

By what mechanism do these antigen–antibody reactions cause disease?
- Hypersensitivity reactions of different types
- Thrombosis
- T-cell activation
- Complement activation

■ Bacteria and spores

What shapes of bacteria are generally recognised and used as part of the classification?

- *Cocci*: small, spherical organisms
- *Bacilli*: straight rod-shaped organisms
- *Vibrios*: comma-shaped organisms
- *Spirilla*: spiral rods that do not bend
- *Spirochaetes*: spiral rods that bend or flex in the middle
- *Actinomycetes*: complex, branching rods (also called higher bacteria)

What is the commonest stain in general use for examining bacteria microscopically?

- Gram stain
  - Most common bacteria
  - Not mycobacteria, which are neither Gram-positive nor Gram-negative as their waxy coat resists staining by the Gram method

What stains are used in a Gram stain?

Crystal violet with a safranin counterstain. Gram-positive organisms are blue-violet and Gram-negative organisms are pink-red as the crystal violet is washed out.

Name one other stain in common microbiological use.

Ziehl–Neelsen stain for mycobacteria; the carbol-fuchsin stain is heated to force it into the micro-organism. The slide is then washed with acid or alcohol. Mycobacteria retain the stain because of waxes in the cell wall; the stain is washed out of other organisms.

What structures may be present as part of the anatomy of a micro-organism?

- *Capsules*: polysaccharides that coat the walls of the organism and contributes to virulence by resisting phagocytosis, found in *Streptococcus pneumoniae, Klebsiella pneumoniae, Bacillus anthracis, Haemophilus influenzae* and meningococci. Capsulate organisms, in particular, cause infections in patients who have had a splenectomy
- *Flagellae*: for locomotion
- *Fimbriae*: thinner and shorter than flagella, used for adhesion
- *Spores*: protect against dehydration, heat and chemicals, and permit survival if starvation threatens; found in *Bacillus* and *Clostridia* spp.

■ Benign neoplasms leading to the death of a patient

How could a benign neoplasm cause disease that leads to the death of a patient?

- Life-threatening obstruction
  - Direct
    - Biliary and pancreatic obstruction by adenoma of the biliary or pancreatic ducts
    - Obstruction to CSF flow in the CNS by meningioma and ependymoma
  - Indirect
    - Intussusception from a polyp in the caecum, transverse colon or sigmoid colon as the intussuscipiens
- Other pressure effects
  - Venous obstruction by leiomyoma of uterus
  - Retrosternal follicular adenoma of thyroid causing venous obstruction
  - Non-functioning pituitary adenoma compressing adjacent gland
- Severe haemorrhage
  - From a large bowel or endometrial polyp
  - From a capillary haemangioma in an infant
- Infection leading to septicaemia
  - Ulcerated large bowel polyps
  - Infection of the biliary system after obstruction by a duct papilloma

- Infarction: torsion of a subserosal fibroid or appendix epiploicae causing abdominal pain and possibly laparotomy
- Fracture through a benign bone tumour such as osteoid osteoma
- Biochemical abnormalities that are life-threatening
  - Eutopic hormone secretion
    - Pituitary adenoma secreting growth hormone (hGH), adrenocorticotropic hormone (ACTH) and thyroid-stimulating hormone (TSH) (prolactin [PRL], follicle-stimulating hormone [FSH] and luteinising hormone [LH] secreting adenomas are unlikely to threaten life)
    - Adrenal adenoma secreting cortisol or aldosterone (testosterone is unlikely to threaten life)
    - Ovarian granulosa cell tumour or thecoma secreting oestrogens and causing endometrial carcinoma
    - Parathyroid adenoma secreting parathyroid hormone
    - Phaeochromocytoma secreting catecholamines
  - Ectopic secretion is usually a feature of malignant tumours, though some biologically benign pancreatic islet cell tumours can secrete ectopic polypeptide hormones such as gastrinoma
  - Potassium and protein loss from large bowel polyps
- Other circulation abnormalities that can be dangerous: polycythaemia, associated with very large uterine leiomyomas
- *Misdiagnosis*: benign neoplasm or hamartoma being misdiagnosed as carcinoma, with consequent operative and subsequent mortality
- Malignant change

▓ Blastomas

Tumours with the suffix -blastoma tend to have common characteristics. What are they?

These tumours are characteristically rare, occur in childhood, and are composed of small, darkly stained (hyperchromatic) cells which have:

- A high nucleus:cytoplasm ratio
- An aggressive behaviour
- A tendency to metastasise

Give some examples of blastomas.

- *Retinoblastoma*: typically associated with an abnormality of the tumour suppressor gene Rb, both alleles of which have to be abnormal for a cell to be released into continuous proliferation
- *Nephroblastoma*: Wilms' tumour: the extent of tubule formation has a bearing on prognosis
- *Neuroblastoma*: may be adrenal or extra-adrenal but only very rarely arise in the CNS
- *Medulloblastoma*
- *Hepatoblastoma*

Name some blastomas that do not fit the above definition and occur in adults.

- Glioblastoma multiforme (an old-fashioned term for very poorly differentiated glioma)
- Osteoblastoma
- Chondroblastoma

▉ Blood transfusion

A patient is given a very large blood transfusion quickly for an emergency that resulted in massive blood loss. How would you classify the possible complications?

Into immediate and delayed.

What immediate complications may develop?

- Haemolysis from incompatibility to
  - ABO
  - Rhesus
  - White cells
  - Other antigens
- Allergic reactions to exogenous proteins
- Temperature changes
  - Hyperthermia from pyrogens of dead polymorphs, endotoxins
  - Hypothermia from rapid transfusion of chilled blood
- Septicaemia
  - From infusion of infected blood: Gram-negative organisms such as coliforms and *Pseudomonas* spp.
- Metabolic
  - Hyperkalaemia from damaged red cells releasing potassium
  - Hypocalcaemia (though citrate as an anticoagulant is generally no longer used and so hypocalcaemia is now rare: a solution of saline, adenine, glucose and mannitol [SAGM] is used instead)

- Decreased oxygen carrying capacity
- Acidosis
- Circulatory
  - Overtransfusion, hypervolaemia causing pulmonary oedema
  - Hypotension because of incompatibility
  - Air embolism
- Bleeding diathesis
  - Transfusion blood may be deficient in platelets and clotting factors, especially factor VII

What delayed complications may develop?

- Sensitisation to foreign antigens
  - Delayed haemolytic reactions from weak immuno-globulins that are undetected and gradually have an effect
- Impaired ability to reject transplanted organs such as renal transplants, especially if repeated transfusions are given
- Infection (in unscreened donor blood) from
  - Hepatitis B, hepatitis C
  - HIV
  - Cytomegalovirus (CMV)
  - Syphilis
  - Malaria
  - Septicaemia from bacteria in blood infected post-donation, or from deficiency in aseptic technique of connection of giving-set, from *Staphylococcus aureus* or coliforms
- Iron overload

■ Bone tumours

What is the commonest malignant neoplasm in bone?
Metastatic carcinoma especially from breast, prostate, lung, kidney and thyroid, in that order of frequency.

What is the commonest malignant neoplasm arising in bone?
Myeloma. About half of all primary malignant neoplasms arising in bone are myelomas.

What is the commonest malignant neoplasm of bone?
Osteosarcoma. About 25% of all primary malignant neoplasms of bone are osteosarcomas, 15% are chondrosarcomas and the remaining 10% are the rest.

What non-neoplastic lesions arise in bone?
- Bone cysts (a loose term including non-cystic but radiolucent lesions)
  - Simple or unicameral bone cyst
  - Aneurysmal bone cyst
  - Maxillomandibular cysts: periapical, radicular, dentigerous, gingival, traumatic, odontogenic and other specific names
  - So-called cysts subchondrally in osteoarthritis and Paget's disease of bone
- Fibrous dysplasia of bone: a patch of woven bone that cannot be replaced by lamellar bone. Polyostotic dysplasia with endocrine abnormalities in Albright's syndrome

- Non-ossifying fibroma
- Neurofibroma
- Osteochondroma, a hamartoma of which the principal abnormality is in the cartilage cap rather than the bone below

What benign neoplasms arise in bone?

- Osteoma
  - *Osteoid osteoma*: radiolucent area, never affects the skull
  - *Ivory osteoma*: radiodense area, only affects the skull
- Osteoblastoma
- Osteoclastoma (in 90% of cases – the rest behave aggressively)
- Chondroblastoma
- Chondroma
  - Solitary (commonest)
  - Multiple
    - Ollier's disease, in which there is usually a unilateral distribution
    - Maffucci's syndrome, with multiple hemangiomas
    - Chondromatosis, with multiple enchondromas and osteochondromas
- Intraosseous lipoma (which might not be a true neoplasm)

■ Bowel organisms

What is the commonest organism in the large bowel?
Bacteroides fragilis

What is a commensal and a transit organism in the large bowel?
- Commensal organism
  - A micro-organism normally found in large numbers in the large bowel that in normal circumstances causes no disease in the host and protects the host from colonisation by pathogenic organisms.
- Transit organism
  - A micro-organism that is occasionally found in small numbers in the large bowel as it traverses the alimentary system; most people suffer no disease but immunodeficient patients might. Microbiology usually do not report organisms found in small numbers that are known to be possible transit organisms.

Give examples of commensals and transit organisms in the large bowel.
- Commensals
  - *Bacteroides* spp.
  - *Escherichia coli*
  - *Enterococcus* spp. such as *faecalis* and *faecium*
- Transit organisms (selected for by exposure to antibiotics, especially cephalosporins)
  - *Clostridium difficile*

- *Candida albicans*
- *Pseudomonas aeruginosa*

Under what circumstances can apparently commensal organisms in the gastrointestinal tract (GIT) cause disease in the intact intestine?

- Immunodeficient patients
  - Congenitally immunodeficient patients
  - Iatrogenically immunosuppressed patients
  - Patients with acquired immunodeficiency such as those with leukaemia, myeloma
- Patients with immunodeficiency and a complicating factor
  - Patients with diabetes mellitus
  - Patients with carcinoma on chemotherapy
- When an apparent commensal becomes pathogenic: *Clostridium difficile*
- Others
  - Impaired perfusion
  - Breach of the wall, such as in diverticulitis
  - Hypotension
  - Primary vascular diseases of the GIT

■ Breast cancer I: epidemiology

How common is breast cancer in the UK?

- The age-standardised incidence and mortality in the USA and the UK are the highest in the world
- The Netherlands also has high incidence
- Japan has a very low incidence for a developed country
- Poorer 5 year survival rates in the UK than in any other European country

How does the incidence of breast cancer change with time and geography?

- Doubles with each decade of increased age until the menopause, when the rate of increase falls sharply
- Is increasing slowly particularly among elderly women by about 1–2% a year
- Lobular carcinoma has increased sharply over the last 20 years; the incidence of ductal carcinoma has remained constant
- The incidence of breast cancer in migrants assumes the rate in the host country within one or two generations

What are the risk factors for the development of breast cancer?

- High-risk factors for referral
  - Age: 50–64 years for screening, 35–50 years if symptomatic for triple assessment
  - Cancer in other breast: invasive or in-situ carcinoma
  - Previous breast disease such as atypical hyperplasia

- Family history of breast cancer
- Non-specific risk factors
  - Geographical location: developed countries more than developing countries
  - Menarche before age of 11 years
  - Menopause after 54 years: women who have a natural menopause at or after the age of 55 are twice as likely to develop breast cancer as women who have the menopause before the age of 45
  - First full pregnancy in early 40s
  - Higher socioeconomic classes
  - Obesity though only in postmenopausal women
  - Exogenous hormones: oral contraceptives for more than 10 years before the age of 25 years
  - Hormone replacement therapy for more than 10 years
  - Diethylstibestrol exposure

■ Breast cancer II: genetics

What is the prevalence of genetically determined breast cancer?

Up to 10% of breast cancer in Western countries is due to genetic predisposition:

- Breast cancer susceptibility is generally inherited as an autosomal dominant with limited penetrance
- Susceptibility is transmitted through either sex
- Family members can transmit the abnormal gene without developing cancer themselves
- Women most likely to have a genetic mutation are those with
  - Bilateral breast cancer
  - A combination of breast cancer and another epithelial cancer
  - Disease at an early age: most breast cancers that are due to a genetic mutation occur before the age of 65
- Families affected by breast cancer have an excess of ovarian, colonic, prostatic and other cancers attributable to the same inherited mutation

What are the known breast cancer genes?

It is not known how many breast cancer genes there are:

- BRCA1 gene is on the long arm of chromosome 17
- BRCA2 gene is on the long arm of chromosome 13
- These account for most of the very high-risk families – those with four or more breast cancers among close relatives

- Both genes are very large and mutations can occur at almost any position
  - Certain mutations occur at high frequency in defined populations
    - 2% of Ashkenazi Jewish women have specifically-identified mutations
    - Half of all familial breast cancer in Iceland is related to one mutation
- Mutations in two other genes, p53 and PTEN, are associated with familial syndromes (Li-Fraumeni and Cowden's, respectively) that include a high risk of breast cancer

In terms of family relatives with breast cancer, which women are particularly at risk?

A woman who has:

- One first-degree female relative with bilateral breast cancer, or breast and ovarian cancer
- One first-degree female relative with breast cancer diagnosed under the age of 40 years
- One first-degree male relative with breast cancer diagnosed at any age
- Two first- or second-degree relatives with breast cancer diagnosed under the age of 60 years or ovarian cancer at any age on the same side of the family
- Three first- or second-degree relatives with breast and ovarian cancer on the same side of the family

(A first-degree relative is a mother, sister or daughter. A second-degree relative is a grandmother, granddaughter, aunt or niece).

Breast cancer III: histopathology and prognostic factors

What are the main types of breast carcinoma encountered in general surgical practice?

- Invasive ductal carcinoma
- In situ ductal carcinoma
- Invasive lobular carcinoma
- In situ lobular carcinoma
- Paget's disease
- Specific types of breast cancer such as medullary, mucinous and tubular

What factors are of clinical use in predicting the behaviour of breast cancer and its response to treatment?

- General factors
  - Age of the patient
    - Contradictory studies, but increased incidence in node positivity is found in women under 35 years
  - Pregnancy
    - Breast cancer arising in women who are pregnant has a poorer prognosis than in women who are not
    - May be age-related, as young women develop aggressive tumours

- May be because of late-stage presentation as small tumours are less apparent in breasts enlarged in late pregnancy and lactation
- Histological factors
  - Histological type
    - Lobular carcinoma, tubular carcinoma, cribriform carcinoma and papillary carcinoma generally have a better prognosis
  - Histological grade
    - Poorly differentiated tumours are associated with a worse prognosis irrespective of tumour size and LN status
    - Some studies have found that tumours with a poor histological grade have a better response to certain types of chemotherapy
  - Tumour size
    - The size on the histological slide takes precedence over the size measured on the gross specimen
    - The size is taken as the maximum extent of invasive spread, which is evident only microscopically
  - Lymph node involvement
    - The most important single prognostic indicator
    - Disease-free and overall survival rates are inversely proportional to the number of lymph nodes involved
  - Tumour necrosis
    - Associated with an adverse outcome
  - Extent of situ disease
    - A probable prognostic factor for local recurrence

- Molecular markers
  - ER and PR receptors
    - ER/PR positive tumours have a good response rate to chemotherapy compared with negative tumours
  - ERBB-2 (HER 2) positivity
    - A humanized anti-ERBB-2 monoclonal antibody *trastuzumab* (Hercerptin) is effective in some patients with overexpression of ERBB-2

▨ Bruising

What is a bruise?

The common term used for any local extravasation of blood especially in or below the skin and the oral, ocular and other mucosae; less commonly used for bleeding into muscles and below the periosteum.

How are bruises and bruising classified?

- By size
  - Petechial haemorrhages
    - ◆ Very small, usually multiple
  - Purpura
    - ◆ Larger patches, single or multiple
  - Ecchymoses
    - ◆ Large, often single
- By whether the cause is congenital and acquired
- By whether onset is sudden or gradual

List some of the congenital causes of bruising.

- Haemophilia, factor VIII deficiency, sex-linked
- Christmas disease, factor IX deficiency, sex-linked
- von Willebrand's disease
  - A deficiency of von Willebrand's factor (vWf), a protein essential for platelet function and also a factor VIII carrier protein
  - Autosomal dominant with partial penetrance

Classify the acquired causes of bruising.

- Due to direct generalised tissue damage
  - Direct physical trauma
  - Surgery, radiotherapy or chemotherapy
- Due to specific damage to small vessels or fragility of them
  - Cushing's syndrome
  - Drugs such as steroids
  - Scurvy
  - Malaria
  - Allergic reactions
- Due to platelet abnormalities
  - Meningococcal septicaemia
  - Disseminated intravascular coagulopathy (DIC) from carcinoma of the prostate, pancreas, bronchus, and fat embolus
  - Massive blood transfusion
  - Autoimmune disorders such as Idiopathic thrombocytopaenic purpura, Henoch Schonlein purpura
  - Leukaemia
  - Waterhouse–Friderichsen syndrome
  - Other platelet consumption diseases
  - Drugs such as aspirin
- Due to acquired clotting factor abnormalities
  - Drugs such as warfarin and heparin
  - Massive blood transfusion
  - Viral infections

How is a tendency to bruise investigated?

- General
  - Full blood count, film
  - Clotting screen and International Normalised Ratio (INR)
    - Prothrombin time (PT) for extrinsic and common pathway
    - Activated prothrombin time (APTT) for intrinsic and common pathway
- Specific
  - Blood culture
  - Serum cortisol
  - Tumour markers
  - Thick blood films for malaria

Burns of the skin I: agents and classification

What agents cause burns?

- Thermal injury
  - Hot liquids: boiling water, hot fat
  - Frostbite, freezing
- Chemicals
  - Alkalis, acids, irritants
  - Sap of some plants, such as giant hogweed (phytophotodermatosis)
- Electric current
- Ionising radiation
- Friction
- Fire, cinders, sparks

How are skin burns classified?

- As first-, second- or third-degree burns
  - Based on how far into the deeper structures of the skin the tissue injury extends
- As clinically important burns based more on prognosis
  - Superficial partial thickness burn
  - Deep partial thickness burn
  - Full thickness burn
- By risk
  - High risk: children <10 years and adults >50 years
  - Low risk: patients aged 10–50 years

- As minor, moderate or major burns in reference to risk:
  - Minor burns
    - Partial thickness burns involving <15% of body surface area (BSA) in low-risk patients
    - Partial thickness burns involving 10% in high-risk patients
    - Full thickness burns of <2% without other injuries
  - Moderate burns
    - Partial thickness burns of 15–25% BSA in low-risk patients
    - 10–20% BSA in high-risk patients
    - Full thickness burns of 3–10% BSA without other injuries
  - Major burns
    - Partial thickness burns >25% BSA in low-risk patients
    - Full thickness burns >10% BSA in anyone
    - Burns involving hands, face, feet or perineum
    - Burns involving major joints of a limb
    - Burns complicated by
      - Fractures
      - Inhalation injury
      - Electrical burns

How are the tissue changes in and around a burn classified?

There are classically three zones of a burn:

- *Zone of coagulation*: non-viable tissue at the centre of the burn in which the proteins and other components have coagulated

- *Zone of ischaemia or stasis*: tissues deep and peripheral to the coagulated centre are not devitalised at first but microvascular injury can cause necrosis after some days if untreated
- *Zone of hyperaemia*: peripheral tissues are not injured by the burn, remain viable, and develop vasodilatation because of release of inflammatory mediators

How is the extent of burns determined?

By the percentage of body area involved, estimated by the Rule of 9s:

- Head and neck: 9%
- Upper limbs: each 9%
- Front of thorax and abdomen: 18%
- Back of thorax and abdomen: 18%
- Lower limbs: each 18%
- Genitalia: 1%

How does the Rule of 9s differ in children?

The head is proportionately much bigger in young children and the lower limbs smaller, so the percentages are reversed, that is, head and neck in children: 18%, lower limbs: each 9%.

The estimation is rough but better than before the correction.

■ Burns of the skin II: clinical aspects

What are the characteristics of a first-degree burn?

A first-degree burn involves only the epidermis:

- The site is red, dry, swollen and peels after a few days
- Pain usually lasts 48 to 72 hours and then subsides
- There are no blisters
- Long-term tissue damage is rare
- There may be an increase or decrease in skin colour
- It usually heals within a week without treatment
- Treatment includes
    - Cold compresses
    - Lotion or ointments
    - Aspirin
    - (Not usually bandaged)

What are the characteristics of a second-degree burn?

A second-degree burn involves the epidermis and the dermis:

- The site is deep red, blistered, wet, shiny and swollen
- Some or all of the burn might be white or irregularly discoloured
- Pain lasts for more than a week
- Long-term scarring is possible
- Superficial second-degree burns usually heal in about three weeks, as long as the wound is clean and protected
- Deep second-degree burns may take longer than three weeks to heal
- Treatment includes
    - Antibiotic ointments

- Dressing changes once or twice a day, depending on severity
- Daily cleaning of the wound, which may require analgesia
- Systemic antibiotics in some case

What are the characteristics of a third-degree burn?

A third-degree burn destroys the epidermis and dermis and so by definition extends into the subcutis or even further:

- The site is white, or dry and leathery, or charred and black
- There is no sensation – the nerve endings are destroyed
- Large burns heal slowly and poorly even with surgical intervention
- The epidermis and dermis are destroyed and so new skin will not grow from below
- Treatment includes
  - Early cleaning and debridement
  - Intravenous fluids containing electrolytes
  - Antibiotics intravenously or by mouth
  - Antibiotic ointments or creams
  - A warm, humid environment for the burn
  - Nutritional supplements and a high-protein diet
  - Analgesics
  - Skin grafts

What are the complications of burns other than the direct tissue damage caused?

- Compartment syndrome
- Renal damage from myoglobinaemia
- Protein loss
- Laryngeal oedema

■ Calcification

How do you classify calcification in the human body?
Orthotopic and heterotopic. Heterotopic calcification is divided into metastatic, dystrophic and age related (which may be dystrophic in some cases).

Where in the body does calcification occur normally (orthotopic calcification)?
- Bones and cartilage
- Teeth
- Otoliths

What is the definition of metastatic calcification? Give examples.
Metastatic calcification occurs as the result of hypercalcaemia with deposition:
- Around the gastric glands
- Around the renal tubules (nephrocalcinosis)
- In the walls of the alveoli of the lungs

What do each of these sites have in common?
They all excrete acid:
- The stomach secretes HCl
- The kidney excretes H^+
- The lung excretes CO_2

What is the definition of dystrophic calcification?

Calcification in dead or damaged tissues in the presence of a normal circulating calcium concentration:

- Tuberculous focus in the lung
- Atheroma
- Scars
- Paracytic cysts such as cysticercosis
- Damaged muscle

Calculi

What is the definition of a calculus?
An abnormal mass formed of precipitated solid material in a duct or bladder (the definition makes no mention of calcium).

What are the five commonest sites of calculus formation?
- Prostatic ducts (by far the commonest; most transurethral resection of the prostate (TURP) and retropubic prostatectomy specimens have calculi)
- Biliary, especially gall bladder
- Urinary system
- Pancreatic ducts
- Salivary gland ducts

What are the principles of calculus formation?
- Primary
  - Increased colloid content of the secreted fluid
- Secondary
  - Nidus formation
  - Decreased solvent
  - Change in pH
  - Stasis of fluid

What may form a nidus?
- Focal papillary necrosis in the kidney
- Infection leading to tissue damage
- Desquamated cells
- Inspissated secretions

What are biliary and urinary calculi composed of?

- Biliary tract
  - Primary
    - Cholesterol
    - Pigment (calcium bilirubinate)
    - Calcium carbonate
  - Secondary
    - Mixed
- Urinary tract
  - Primary
    - Oxalate
    - Urate
    - Cystine
    - Xanthine
  - Secondary
    - Calcium phosphate
    - Calcium carbonate
    - Magnesium ammonium phosphate

What are the complications of calculi?

- Obstruction owing to impaction of the calculus in the ureter or cystic duct causing severe pain
- Haemorrhage especially in the urinary tract
- Stricture because of irritation by the calculus in the ureter
- Perforation with migration of the calculus into an adjacent organ such as in gall stone ileus
- Infection in the renal pelvis
- Squamous metaplasia in the bladder
- Malignant change in the bladder in long-standing cases

■ *Candida* infection

What organism causes candidiasis (candidosis)?
There are over 200 species in the *Candida* genus, the commonest human pathogen being *Candida albicans*.

How is *candida* infection diagnosed?
- Microscopy of sputum, skin swab or other material
- Culture on Sabaraud's medium
- Antigen detection in serum, urine or other fluid
- Antibody detection in serum
- Finding increased concentration of arabinitol, a metabolite of *candida*, in serum (not routine in UK)

What sites are affected by candidiasis?
- Mucous membranes
  - Vagina and cervix
  - Mouth
  - Pharynx
  - Oesophagus
- Skin folds especially in intertrigo
- Face and scalp in chronic mucocutaneous candidiasis
- Lower respiratory tract
- Urinary tract
- Septicaemia with localisation in eye, endocardium, meninges, kidney, bone marrow

What groups of patients are likely to be affected?
Patients with:
- Diabetes mellitus

- Immunodeficiency
  - AIDS
  - Congenital
  - Drug induced, such as by steroids and cytotoxic agents
  - Debilitation
  - Malignant disease especially when widespread
- Leukaemia, myeloma
- Diseases requiring long-term antibiotic therapy

What other less common fungal diseases may patients suffer from?

- *Cryptococcus neoformans*
- *Malassezia furfur*
- Dermatophytes
- *Torulopsis glabrata*
- *Aspergillus fumigatus* (the commonest human pathogen in this genus), *Aspergillus flavus* and *Aspergillus niger*
- *Pneumocystis carinii* (now called *Pneumocystis jiroveci*)

■ Carcinogenesis I: chemical carcinogenesis

How are chemical carcinogens classified?

- Into remote, proximate and ultimate carcinogens.

What is a remote carcinogen?

- A precursor of a carcinogenic agent that might be found in food, the environment, exposure to certain chemicals and physical agents, and infective organisms.

What is a proximate carcinogen?

- The metabolite or metabolites of a remote carcinogen that have some carcinogenic potential but may be modified further in the body into an ultimate carcinogen.

What is an ultimate carcinogen?

- The active carcinogen that interacts with DNA and causes cancer.

How do chemical carcinogens act?

- If they are hydrocarbons they form epoxides, charged molecules that form covalent bonds with DNA, RNA and proteins.

Give an example of a remote – proximate – ultimate carcinogen sequence.

- β-naphthylamine is used by rubber and dye workers. It is not intrinsically carcinogenic: experimentally it can be washed into the bladder and retained with no deleterious effects. It may be considered to be a remote carcinogen.

- When ingested, β-naphthylamine is absorbed through the small bowel and metabolised in the liver by hydroxylation to an actively carcinogenic agent (there is no good evidence that β-naphthylamine causes gastric carcinoma).
- In the liver, the carcinogen is conjugated with glucuronic acid and made water soluble (there is no evidence that the incidence of hepatocellular carcinoma is increased in rubber and dye workers). The conjugated molecule is a proximate carcinogen.
- The conjugated carcinogen is excreted by the kidneys and stored in urine in the bladder for a variable period.
- The problem arises because normal urothelium and micro-organisms causing cystitis secrete glucuronidase, which digests the protective glucuronic acid and releases the ultimate carcinogen into the bladder.
- This results in the development of transitional cell carcinoma.

■ Carcinogenesis II: agents

Name some chemical carcinogens other than β-naphthylamine.

- Nitrosamines and nitrosamides, nitrates and nitrites.
  - Nitrosamides do not require metabolism to become carcinogenic.
- Alkylating agents such as busulphan and cyclo-phosphamide cause leukaemia and lymphoma.
- Aflatoxin from *Aspergillus flavus* causes hepatocellular carcinoma and liver cell necrosis by affecting the *p53* gene.

What occupational carcinogens are important surgically?

- β-naphthylamine: bladder carcinoma
- Asbestos: squamous cell carcinoma of bronchus, mesothelioma of pleura and peritoneum
- Vinyl chloride monomer: angiosarcoma of liver
- Hardwood sawdust: adenocarcinoma of nasal spaces
- Nickel: carcinoma of bronchus, larynx
- Arsenic: carcinoma of bronchus, skin

What is an initiator in the development of cancer?

- An initiator changes the DNA in a cell so that the progeny of the cell becomes abnormal.
- It does not necessarily cause neoplasia though may do so in large doses.

What is a promoter?

- A promoter affects normal cells and initiated cells and causes changes that lead to altered gene expression. Only in initiated cells with abnormal DNA does the altered gene expression result in a preneoplastic or a neoplastic cell.

- More than one promoter event may be necessary to induce neoplasia.
- Hormones may be considered to be promoters in human carcinoma.

■ Carcinoma and sarcoma

Define carcinoma.
A malignant tumour composed of epithelial cells.

(*Not* a malignant tumour of ectodermally-derived cells. The embryological origin of the epithelial cells is immaterial. The kidney, ovary, fallopian tube and endometrium are all derived from mesoderm but nonetheless develop carcinoma.)

Define sarcoma.
A malignant tumour composed of connective tissue cells.

(As above, named for what the tumour is composed of and not where it arises. The tissue of origin is immaterial. Osteosarcoma of the breast and of the buttock are well recognised.)

How is carcinoma typed?
Into four main types:
- Squamous cell carcinoma
- Adenocarcinoma
- Transitional cell carcinoma
- Undifferentiated (anaplastic) carcinoma

Carcinomas of specialised cells are named for those cells, such as:
- Melanoma
- Basal cell carcinoma
- Hepatocellular carcinoma

How is sarcoma typed?

By the tissue that forms the greatest volume of the tumour or that has the worse or worst prognosis.

Give examples of sarcomas.

- Osteosarcoma
- Chrondrosarcoma
- Fibrosarcoma
- Liposarcoma

How are carcinoma and sarcoma graded?

Usually into well differentiated, moderately differentiated, poorly differentiated (and undifferentiated if there is no attempt at recognisable tissue formation).

What are the prognostic indicators that can be derived from the histological appearance of a malignant tumour?

- Tumour type (the cell type accounting for the tumour; there may be mixed cell types)
- Tumour grade (the differentiation of a tumour into well, moderately and poorly differentiated)
- Tumour stage (the extent of spread of a tumour)
- Whether the tumour extends to excision margins
- Whether there are associated features of prognostic importance such as dysplasia, viral infection, evidence of the effects of radiotherapy and chemotherapy, hormone secretion, involvement of vessels or vital structures

■ Cell cycle

Draw a simple version of the normal cell cycle and label the parts.

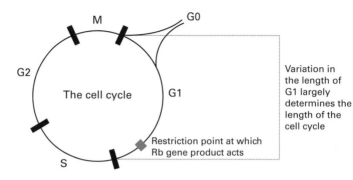

What do the terms mean?

- G1 is gap 1. The variation in the length of a cell's cycle is determined mostly by the length of time it spends in G1 (and to a much lesser extent in G2). If the cell cycle is permitted to advance beyond the restriction point, the cell must complete the cycle and undergo mitosis. The retinoblastoma gene Rb product acts at the restriction point
- S is the synthesis phase in which cell wall, cytoplasmic and nuclear proteins are formed
- G2 is the second gap phase, the length of which varies slightly in different cells and among species
- M is the phase of mitosis
- G0 is when the cell enters a resting phase before re-entering the cycle

What agents control progression around the cycle?

- Cyclins
- Cyclin-dependent kinases (CDKs)
- p53, p27 and p21 that inhibit CDKs
- Rb and related genes which hold the cell in G1

Which factors stimulate growth in inflammation and repair?

- Epidermal growth factor (EGF) from epithelial cells:
  - Homology with *c-erb*B-2 gene product
- Platelet-derived growth factor (PDGF) from α granules in platelets and from macrophages:
  - Homology with *c-sis* gene product
- Fibroblast growth factors
- Cytokines such as insulin-like growth factor I and tumour necrosis factor
- Transforming growth factor α, which is very similar to EGF

Cell damage by ionising radiation

How is ionising radiation classified?
- *Electromagnetic*: X-rays, γ-rays, cosmic radiation
- *Particulate*: α-particles, β-particles, electron capture as a result of β emission

How is cell damage by radiation classified?
- Direct DNA damage
  - From thymidine–thymidine (TT) dimers and other cross linkages
  - From free radicals
  - (Cells are most sensitive during G2 and M, and least sensitive during S)
- Indirect DNA damage
  - Protein damage
  - Damage to cell membrane lipopolysaccharide
  - Enzyme damage

What dose of whole-body radiation causes symptoms?

Rads	Effect
100,000	Death within minutes
10,000	Death within hours from central nervous system (CNS) effects
1,000	Death perhaps in weeks from pancytopaenia and ulceration in the small and large bowel
100	Nausea and vomiting

Which tissues are radiosensitive, intermediate and radioresistant?

- *Radiosensitive*: bone marrow, gonads, growing cartilage and bone, lens of eye, bowel, thyroid, pituitary, kidney, heart, lung, liver, brain, skin
- *Intermediate*: adult cartilage and bone, mucosa of mouth, oesophagus and bladder
- *Radioresistant*: uterus and vagina, adrenal gland, pancreas

■ Chromosomal abnormalities I: classification

How many chromosomes are there in a normal cell?
- 0, 23, 46, 92, any multiple of 46 – all can be normal
- Most cells have 46 chromosomes, 44 autosomes and 2 sex chromosomes
- Cells with 23 chromosomes are haploid. They are found in gonads as late spermatocytes, spermatids, spermatozoa and oocytes
- Cells with 92 are tetraploid cells that have duplicated their chromosomal material before division
- Normal cells with no chromosomes are erythrocytes
- Normal cells with high multiples of 46 are multinucleate, such as osteoclasts and muscle cells

How are chromosome abnormalities classified?
Abnormalities of:
- Autosome structure
- Autosome number
- Autosome location
- Sex chromosome structure
- Sex chromosome number
- Sex chromosome location – for example, Y-chromosomal material may be found on several other chromosomes

What are the two principal types of abnormality of chromosome structure?
- *Translocations*: parts of chromosomes are transposed onto others: may be balanced, when material is reciprocally

transferred and so the total is unaffected, or unbalanced when material is gained or lost

- *Deletions*: loss of chromosomal material of an amount or type that is compatible with development of a living organism. Deletion of material from both ends of a chromosome with fusion of the ends results in ring chromosome formation

■ Chromosomal abnormalities II: DNA ploidy

What does DNA ploidy refer to?
The amount of DNA in a cell. This may or may not correlate with chromosome number.

In terms of ploidy, what is a normal cell?
- A normal cell (other than a red cell) is haploid, diploid, tetraploid or occasionally polyploid.
- Abnormal cells may be aneuploid, either by gaining chromosomal material in odd amounts or by gaining or losing entire chromosomes.

What do the terms monosomy, trisomy and triploidy mean?
- -somy refers to single chromosomes: -ploidy refers to sets of 23 chromosomes
- Loss of one of a pair of chromosomes is called *monosomy*. This is usually incompatible with life, though women with Turner's syndrome could be considered to be monosomic for a sex chromosome
- An increase to three of one type of chromosome is called *trisomy* and is a relatively common occurrence, as in Down's syndrome
- Polyploidy is when there are entire extra sets of all 23 chromosomes, the commonest being triploidy with three

sets giving 69 chromosomes. This is incompatible with life after a few weeks gestation

How is DNA ploidy measured?

By a variety of methods. Flow cytometry is a common method; DNA densitometry is less widely used.

■ Chromosomal abnormalities III: Down's syndrome

What are the surgically important complications of people with Down's syndrome?

- Congenital heart defects: persistent ductus arteriosus (PDA), ventricular septal defect (VSD) and atrial septal defect (ASD)
- Increased risk of neoplasia
- Increased susceptibility to infections
- Increased risk of glue ear
- Cosmetic reasons possibly, such as tongue reduction, revision of epicanthic folds – the ethics and desirability of these are debated

What is the chromosomal abnormality that is present and how may this arise?

Three copies of chromosome 21 material (one-and-a-half times the normal amount) in all or some cells.

Can occur by:

- Non-disjunction (commonest: affects mothers over 40 years)
- Translocation (rare: affects young mothers who have, or whose partners have, a balanced translocation of chromosome 21 and so are normal)
- Mosaicism

How may non-disjunction cause trisomy 21?

- Almost all people with Down's syndrome have cells that all have trisomy 21. The extra copy is the result of non-disjunction of a gamete during meiosis – one daughter cell receives both copies of chromosome 21 and the other none. The gamete without chromosome 21 is non-viable. When the gamete with the extra chromosome 21 is fertilised by a normal gamete from the other parent, three copies are present in the resulting ovum.

- Non-disjunction may occur in both sexes: Down's syndrome children are more prevalent when the father as well as the mother is older, though in practice this applies only to men over 70 years.

How can translocation cause trisomy 21?

- Translocation accounts for a small proportion of cases. Translocation of chromosome 21 material onto another autosome such as chromosome 14 or chromosome 22 can mean that the mother or father is phenotypically normal – they have the normal amount of chromosome 21, though it is in the wrong place because of translocation. One chromosome 21 is absent and so this is a *balanced* translocation.

- One-quarter of the affected parent's gametes will have two copies of the genetic material of chromosome 21 (one as the definitive chromosome 21 and the other translocated to chromosome 14 or 22). When this joins with a normal gamete from the other parent, an ovum with three copies of chromosome 21 results.

How may mosaicism cause trisomy 21?

- About 1 in 100 cases of Down's syndrome are due to mosaicism. The ovum has a normal complement of chromosomes but there is non-dysjunction after the blastocyst starts to develop. Only a proportion of cells will be affected.

Somatic cell in a
normal person

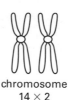

chromosome
14 × 2

chromosome
21 × 2

Somatic cell in a
normal person
with a balanced
translocation

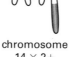

chromosome
14 × 2+

chromosome
21 × 1

Gametes

Normal

Not viable –
missing
too much
chromosomal
material

After fertilisation,
results in balanced
translocation –
carrier for Down's
syndrome in the
next generation

After fertilisation,
results in trisomy
21 – translocation
form of Down's
syndrome

C | **Chromosomal abnormalities III: Down's syndrome**

■ Chromosomal abnormalities IV: sex chromosomes

What abnormalities of sex chromosomes are of surgical importance?

- Turner's syndrome and Kleinfelter's syndrome are the two most important.

What is the abnormality and the phenotype in a woman with Turner's syndrome?

X0 (Y0 is fatal as there is insufficient genetic material for life):

- Coarctation of the aorta
- Webbing of neck
- Wide carrying angle
- Shield chest
- Short stature
- Streak ovaries and aplasia of uterus. The ovaries may contain germ cells – women with Turner's syndrome can develop dysgerminoma
- No learning disability

As one of the two X-chromosomes in each cell in a normal woman is inactivated by lyonisation, resulting in cells with only one active X-chromosome, why are women with Turner's syndrome abnormal?

- Lyonisation is *incomplete* inactivation of an X-chromosome.

What is the abnormality in Kleinfelter's syndrome?

- XXY, presence of an extra sex chromosome. As the Y-chromosome with its *sry* sex determining region induces testicular development and a male phenotype, it is generally considered that the extra chromosome is one of the Xs. Rarely men with Kleinfelter's syndrome are XXXY or XXXXY.

What is the phenotype of a man with Kleinfelter's syndrome?

- Tall stature from longer than normal lower limbs
- Small external genitalia and infertility
- Gynaecomastia (with the risk of breast cancer the same as that of a woman)
- Female distribution of body hair
- No learning disability except in rare cases

What are hermaphroditism and pseudohermaphroditism?

- True hermaphroditism is when a person has both ovarian and testicular tissue, either together in the same gonad or as a testis and ovary on different sides.
- The karyotype is usually XX though a Y-chromosome may be found in some patients. When a Y-chromosome is present there is a high risk of the patient developing teratoma, dysgerminoma and other neoplasms.
- Pseudohermaphroditism is when the gonads reflect the genotype but the phenotype is mismatched. For example, a boy may have normal chromosomes and testes but ambiguous genitalia because of androgen insensitivity or deficiency in conversion of testosterone to dihydro-testosterone; a chromosomally normal girl may develop clitoromegaly from congenital adrenal hyperplasia.

■ Chromosomal abnormalities V: autosomal dominant

What does *autosomal dominant* mean?

An autosomal dominant condition is one in which a single copy of an abnormal autosome confers the disease:

- One parent must be affected (assuming that this is not a spontaneous mutation)
- Half of the children would be affected (this is actuarial: all or none could be affected, and this assumes that only one parent is normal)
- Male and female children have an equal chance of being affected

Give some examples and say why they are of surgical importance.

- Familial adenomatous polyposis
  - several chromosomal abnormalities
  - affects mucosal cells in the GIT
  - results in adenomatous polyps
  - adenocarcinoma arises in almost all cases
- Polycystic kidney
  - Presents in adult life
  - Bilaterally affected kidneys develop large cysts and chronic renal failure ensues
  - Associated with berry aneurysm of the circle of Willis and polycystic disease of the liver, pancreas and spleen
  - Occasionally associated with aneurysms elsewhere such as the aorta, diverticula of the small and large bowel, and ovarian cysts

- Achondroplasia
  - Abnormal development of bones formed on a cartilage matrix
  - Increased risk of fractures
  - Increased incidence of osteoarthritis
- Marfan's syndrome
  - Connective tissue deficit
  - Heart valve abnormalities leading to cardiac failure
  - Increased risk of aortic dissection
  - Increased risk of subluxation of the lens of the eye
- Spherocytosis
  - Congenital cause of haemolytic anaemia
  - Increased risk of gallstones
  - Treated by splenectomy

What does autosomal co-dominance mean?

- In most cells, only one of the pair of a particular gene is active and makes all of the gene product
- Some genes act as a pair to make half of the gene product each
- An abnormality of one of a pair of co-dominant genes knocks out half of the gene function but not all of it. Examples include:
- Some red cell enzymes and haemoglobins
  - Sickle cell disease
  - Acid phosphatase, adenylate kinase
- Some plasma proteins: haptoglobulins
- Some cell surface antigens: human leucocyte antigen (HLA)

Chromosomal abnormalities V: autosomal dominant

■ Chromosomal abnormalities VI: autosomal recessive

What does *autosomal recessive* mean?

An autosomal recessive condition is one in which both copies of an abnormal gene must be present before the disease develops:

- Both parents must have at least one copy of the abnormal gene: they could be heterozygous carriers, or one could be a carrier and one homozygous, or very rarely both parents could be homozygous if the disease carries no risk of infertility or death before puberty
- When a heterozygous carrier has a normal partner, half of the children would be expected to be carriers
- When two carriers have children, one in four children would be expected to have the disease, one in four will be normal and two in four will be carriers

Give some examples and say why they are of surgical importance.

- Cystic fibrosis
  - Abnormality of chromosome 7q causing chloride transportation deficit
  - Susceptibility to infections
  - Tendency to develop
    - Bronchiectasis
    - Pancreatitis
    - Cirrhosis
    - Intestinal obstruction from meconium ileus

- α_1 Antitrypsin deficiency
  - Better called *protease-inhibitor deficiency*
  - Most people in the world are normal and are homozygous for the M variant
  - Some normal people are heterozygous MZ
  - Affected patients are either homozygous for the Z form (ZZ) or are hemizygous for Z (Z−) and lack one allele
  - Tendency to develop emphysema, hepatitis and cirrhosis
- Congenital adrenal hyperplasia
  - Absence of 21 hydroxylase resulting in
    - Virilisation of female fetuses and infants and so ambiguous genitalia
    - Salt loss
    - Hypotension
  - Absence of 11 hydroxylase resulting in
    - Virilisation of female fetuses and infants
    - Ambiguous genitalia
    - Salt retention

◼ Chromosomal abnormalities VII: X-linked

What does *X-linked* (or *sex-linked*) mean?

A disorder that is caused by an abnormality on the X-chromosome (the very small Y-chromosome carries little genetic message and diseases related to its absence (Turner's syndrome) are rare)

- Diseases that are recessive and sex-linked affect males almost exclusively
- Female carriers are normal (if they were homozygous for the abnormal gene they would be considered to be affected rather than normal)

If a female carrier married a normal man (the commonest eventuality)

- Half of all sons would be affected: this could be all or none but actuarially half will be affected
- Half of the daughters would be expected to be carriers
- Sons who are unaffected by the disease cannot be carriers

All of the daughters of a father who is affected will be carriers. (*Not* actuarially but obligatorily.)

Give some examples.

Haemophilia and Christmas disease

- Abnormal bleeding because of deficiency or abnormality of factors VIII and IX
- Haemarthroses
- Intramuscular haematomas

- Haemorrhage at surgical operation
- Common cause of death is AIDS from infected blood transfusions

von Willebrand's disease is autosomal dominant. It is not intrinsically a clotting factor deficiency but a deficiency of von Willebrand factor (vWf) which results in defective adhesion of platelets and a prolonged bleeding time (vWf carries factor VIII in the plasma and so deficiency results in low factor VIII)

- Glucose-6-phosphate dehyrogenase deficiency
  - Haemolysis caused by drugs such as sulphonamides, antimalarials, nitrofurantoin and sulphones for leprosy
- Fragile X syndrome
  - Commonest cause for inherited severe learning disability
  - Long narrow head, long face, very large ears
  - Very large testes that could present a surgical diagnostic problem unless recognised
- Red-green colour blindness
  - Commonest X-linked disorder, affects one in ten men
  - Of surgical importance when a surgeon is colour blind and unaware of the fact
  - Commoner in consultant histopathologists than would be expected by chance

■ Clostridia I: classification

How are Clostridia described in terms of staining and cultural characteristics?

Gram-positive, spore bearing, exotoxin-producing bacteria that are anaerobes with varying degrees of resistance to the toxic effects of oxygen. Oxygen causes free radical formation in all cells and anaerobes have no or few defence mechanisms. Clostridia are saprophytyes – they live in soil and have spores to protect them from dehydration.

What are the commonly encountered types of Clostridia?

There are over 150 species of Clostridia. The commoner pathogens include:

- *Clostridium botulinum* causes botulism, a rare severe toxic condition in which the exotoxin from *Clostridium botulinum* causes flaccid paralysis with involvement of respiratory muscles.
- *Clostridium perfringens* (formerly *welchii*) causes food poisoning at about 12–18 hours after ingestion of exotoxin, and when the organism causes a deep tissue infection, gas gangrene.
- *Clostridium tetani* causes tetanus, produced by tetanospasmin, a neurotoxin causing muscular spasms and paralysis.
- *Clostridium difficile* causes pseudomembranous colitis. The exotoxin causes cell membrane damage to epithelial

cells with severe ulceration of the large bowel with pyrexia and blood loss. Summit lesions are seen histologically.

Saprophytic clostridia transmitted by deep inoculation of soil organisms include *Clostridium oedematiens* and *Clostridium saprophyticum*.

■ Clostridia II: culture

What cultural and other characteristics do Clostridia have?

- Anaerobes with varying degrees of resistance to oxygen toxicity
- Grow on most anaerobic media
- Saccharolytic types ferment sugars but do not break down proteins
  - Cause gas gangrene
  - Include *Clostridium perfringens, Clostridium oedematiens* and *Clostridium septicum*
- Proteolytic types break down proteins
  - Also involved in gas gangrene, cause the characteristic smell
  - Include *Clostridium histolyticum* and *Clostridium sporogenes*

What toxins are produced by Clostridia?

Exotoxins secreted from the cells which include:

- Neurotoxins which bind to transmitters in nerve endings and other structures
  - Tetanospasmin affects the *central* nervous system
    - Binds to gangliosides at presynaptic inhibitory motor nerve endings
    - Taken up by the axon by endocytosis
    - Blocks release of inhibitory neurotransmitters
    - Causes rigidity and spastic paralysis
  - Botulinus toxin affects the *peripheral* nervous system
    - Blocks motor neurons at neuromuscular junctions
    - Causes weakness or flaccid paralysis

- Enzymes
  - Those that are primarily membrane damaging
    - Lecithinase splits lecithin in cell membranes
    - Haemolysins that damage red cells such as tetanolysin
  - Those that break down intercellular substances
    - Collagenase
    - Hyaluronidase
    - Fibrinolysin

▪ Coagulation cascade

Define coagulation.

Coagulation is a series of enzyme-controlled steps leading to the conversion of soluble plasma proteins (especially fibrinogen) into an insoluble, polymerised deposit which could be a clot or a thrombus.

Which clotting factors are made in the liver?

All of them except calcium, which is Factor IV. Hepatocytes make all of the factors except calcium and factor VIII, the latter being made by endothelial cells (which are also present in the liver).

What are the physiological benefits of the coagulation cascade?

- Limitation of acute (and to a lesser extent chronic) haemorrhage, which is usually venous or capillary rather than arterial
  - External: lacerations, other wounds
  - Internal: intracranial haemorrhage, haemorrhage into a hollow viscus, such as the bladder
- Contribution to localisation of acute infection with abscess formation

The cascade is divided into the intrinsic and the extrinsic systems. What do these terms mean?

- Intrinsic cascade, named because:
  - The components are intrinsic to the blood itself without factors coming from the tissues or elsewhere, relevant to blood clotting in a plain glass tube. Tested by activated

partial thromboplastin time (APTT) (intrinsic and common pathways)

- Extrinsic cascade, named because:
  - Clotting is activated or contributed to by factors provided by tissues usually as a consequence of damage, so not relevant to blood clotting in a plain glass tube. Tested by prothrombin time (PT) (extrinsic and common pathways)

Which clotting factor is particularly calcium dependent?

Factor VII, which is also the factor that decays faster than the others in stored blood, so calcium deficiency affects especially the extrinsic system.

What are the two tests of the coagulation of the blood in common use?

PT and APTT.

What does the PT test?

- Tests the extrinsic and common pathways
- Thromboplastin and calcium are added to the patient's plasma
- The PT is expressed as the International Normalised Ratio

The PT is prolonged in:

- Liver disease
- Vitamin K deficiency
- Warfarin treatment
- Disseminated intravascular coagulopathy

What does the APTT test?

- Tests the intrinsic and common pathways
- Kaolin is added to the patient's plasma

The APTT is prolonged in:

- Liver disease
- Heparin treatment
- Haemophilia and clotting factor deficiencies
- Disseminated intravascular coagulopathy
- Massive blood transfusion
- Patients with lupus anticoagulant

What other tests are there that might be useful?

- The thrombin time:
  - Tests the common pathway
  - Thrombin is added to the patient's plasma
  - Is prolonged in:
    - Heparin treatment
    - Disseminated intravascular coagulopathy
    - Dysfibrinogenaemia
- The bleeding time:
  - Tests platelet function and capillary resistance to bleeding
  - Is prolonged in:
    - Thrombocytopaenia
    - Thrombasthenia
    - Disorders of the vessel wall
    - Haemophilia

How are the bleeding time and the clotting time measured? What other tests of clotting can be derived from the clotting time test?

- *Bleeding time*: the time taken for a lancet puncture hole in an earlobe to stop bleeding. The hole is blotted every 15 seconds with filter paper. The normal bleeding time is

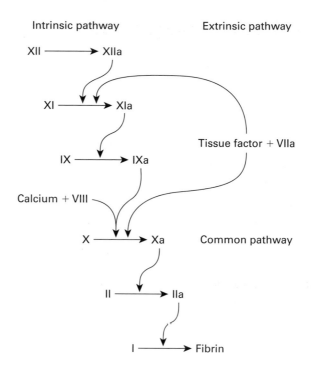

Intrinsic pathway

Extrinsic pathway

XII → XIIa

XI → XIa

IX → IXa

Tissue factor + VIIa

Calcium + VIII

X → Xa   Common pathway

II → IIa

I → Fibrin

3–5 minutes and is principally a measure of platelet function.

- *Clotting time*: the time taken for blood to clot in a glass test tube. The tube is inverted every 60 seconds. The normal clotting time is 4–6 minutes and is a measure of the intrinsic clotting system.
- *Other tests*: clot retraction after the clot has formed in the clotting test is a measure of platelet function.

■ Colorectal cancer I: aetiology

Where in the large bowel does adenocarcinoma arise?

- Prevalence is rectum > sigmoid > caecum > descending > ascending > transverse
- Right-side tumours tend to be polypoid and involve only part of the circumference
- Left-side tumours tend to be annular and constrictive
- Usually well or moderately differentiated adenocarcinoma with no particular differences related to the site of development

List the predisposing factors and associations.

- Colorectal adenoma
  - *Size*: large adenomas have a higher incidence of malignant change
  - *Histological type*: villous papillomas have a higher incidence than tubular adenomas
  - *Differentiation*: severely atypical adenomas have a higher incidence than well-differentiated ones
  - *Age*: increasing incidence with age
- Ulcerative colitis
- Peutz–Jeghers syndrome
- Previous history of polyps or carcinoma
- Family history
  - FAP
  - Hereditary non-polyposis colonic carcinoma (HNPCC)

- Familial colonic cancer syndrome
- Rare genetic abnormalities which predispose to colorectal carcinoma
- Ethnic groups
  - In the USA, Whites more than Blacks; Jews much more than Mormons

In terms of geography, what are the main associations?

- Commoner in Westernised countries than developing countries
- In developed countries, commoner in the west than the east
- May be related to lack of dietary fibre though this is now disputed
- Smoking
- Drinking alcohol
- Lack of exercise

Is there a screening programme for colorectal carcinoma?

- Faecal occult blood test on at least three specimens
- Assay of stools for
  - Protein product of abnormal APC gene
  - Protein product of abnormal BAT26 gene
- Sigmoidoscopy and colonoscopy screening
- Double-contrast barium enema: low sensitivity

■ Colorectal cancer II: genetic aspects

What are the principal patterns of inheritance of colorectal carcinoma?

- Sporadic (no pattern of inheritance)
- FAP
  - Autosomal dominant
  - Accounts for 2% of all colorectal carcinomas
  - Non-classic forms:
    - Attenuated form of FAP (AFAP)
    - Other non-classic forms such as in people of Ashkenazi Jewish descent
- HNPCC
  - Autosomal dominant
  - Accounts for 5% of all colorectal carcinomas
- Familial colorectal carcinoma: runs in families but no gene defect known
- Syndromes such as Lynch II and Li–Fraumeni which include colorectal carcinoma

In the commonest, sporadic type, what genetic abnormalities are characteristic?

- Normal – adenoma – carcinoma sequence involves at least seven major molecular aberration
- Two main pathways
  - Chromosomal instability accounts for 85%

- Aneuploidy and detectable deletions from chromosomes
  - ▲ 5: APC gene, the earliest genetic abnormality
  - ▲ 17: *p53* gene
  - ▲ 18: DCC gene
- Microsatellite instability accounts for 15%
  - Reasonably intact chromosomes but defects in chromosome repair
  - Mutations allowed to persist in repeating DNA units called *microsatellites*

What are the main genetic abnormalities in patients with FAP?

- APC gene abnormality, chromosome 5
  - Codes for a protein important in cell adhesion and signal transmission
  - Over 300 different mutations of the gene are recognised
  - Most are insertions, deletions and nonsense mutations
  - Result in frameshifts and premature stop codons
  - In attenuated FAP, the genetic abnormalities are later in the exon
- *p53* gene abnormality, chromosome 17
- DCC gene abnormality, chromosome 18

And in patients with HNPCC?

- Mutation in one or more of the DNA mismatch repair genes
- Abnormality of:
  - mutS gene on chromosome 2

- mutL gene on chromosome 3
- Other mismatch gene mutations mostly on chromosome 2
- Related to microsatellite instability in many cases

Do all families with a high incidence of colorectal carcinoma fall into the above categories?

- 10–15% of patients with colorectal cancer have affected family members
- No relation with FAP or HNPCC
- No recognisable pattern of inheritance
- No known specific genetic abnormalities
- May be due to:
  - Shared environmental risk factors
  - Genetic factors
  - Chance

■ Colorectal cancer III: staging

What is the minimum criterion for the diagnosis of very early adenocarcinoma of the colorectum?

- There must be penetration of at least one neoplastic gland through the muscularis mucosae into the submucosa

If a neoplastic polyp is confined to the mucosa, is it always benign?

Yes

Does infiltration through the epithelial basement membrane or into the lamina propria of the mucosa have any bearing?

No. An adenocarcinoma in the submucosa will probably show infiltration of the lamina propria but the latter alone does not indicate malignancy. If a neoplastic polyp is confined to the mucosa (including the lamina propria) it is benign.

How is adenocarcinoma of the large bowel staged?

- Dukes' staging (Cuthbert Esquire Dukes 1890–1977, histopathologist)
- TNM staging
- Jass staging

What are the components of Dukes' staging of large bowel cancer? When does one stage become a worse stage?

- Dukes' stage A

- a glandular neoplasm within the wall of the large bowel deep to the mucosa but confined within the outermost aspect of the muscularis propria
- Dukes' stage B
  - a glandular neoplasm extending through the wall of the large bowel beyond the outermost aspect of the muscularis propria but not involving lymph nodes
- Dukes' stage C
  - a glandular neoplasm of the large bowel involving LNs
    - Dukes originally had only stage C. This was later modified to include stage C1 with local LN involvement and stage C2 with distant involvement
    - a carcinoma does not have to extend through A to B to C. An apparently stage A tumour can have LN metastases and so really be stage C

What aspects of the tumour of use in determining its prognosis are not addressed by Dukes' staging method?

- type of growth: pushing or infiltrative
- whether the tumour is completely excised
- whether there is a brisk lymphocytic or histocytic reaction around the tumour cells
- proximity to excision margins
- whether major venous radicles are invaded: this independent variable reduces the prognosis to 15% in 5 years irrespective of Dukes' stage

■ Compartment syndrome

What is meant by a compartment syndrome?

Compartment syndrome arises when the pressure in a closed anatomical space exceeds the perfusion pressure and so compromises the circulation and function of the tissues in the space. The reduction or cessation of circulation may cause temporary or permanent ischaemic damage to muscles and nerves. Crush syndrome is distinct from compartment syndrome though is a cause of it – it occurs when muscle swelling secondary to direct trauma initiates the cycle of events.

Where in the body does a compartment syndrome typically affect?

- The leg (four main compartments)
- The foot (several compartments)
- The forearm (four related compartments). Usually from damage to the brachial artery from a displaced supra-condylar fracture of humerus (von Volkman 1875)
- The abdomen (typically after repair of an abdominal aortic aneurysm)
- The kidney and heart as a *consequence* of the compartment syndrome:
  - Acute tubular necrosis from myoglobin release into the circulation
  - Dysrhythmias from hyperkalaemia

How do you classify the causes of acute compartment syndrome?

- External restriction:
  - Tight splints, dressings or plaster casts
  - Burns with eschar formation
  - Very tight trousers, such as worn by some combat troops
  - Tight fascial closure
  - Tight ski boots
  - Localised external pressure
- Internal increase in the volume in the compartment:
  - Haemorrhage
    - Trauma, surgical operation
    - Anticoagulant drugs, haemophilia
    - Gunshot wounds, other missile injury
  - Fractures
  - Swelling after ischaemia
    - Crush injury
    - Embolisation and embolectomy
  - Snake bite
  - Crush injuries, burns
  - Rhabdomyolysis from viral infections, drug overdose

How is compartment syndrome diagnosed?

On suspicion from symptoms and signs:

- Pain out of proportion to physical signs
- Pain on passive movement
- Pulselessness and palor (too late)

- By measuring pressures – if high or inconclusive, open the compartment fully

What is chronic compartment syndrome?

- An exercise-induced condition characterised by recurrent pain and disability which:
  - Causes symptoms that subside when the exercise is stopped
  - Recurs when the activity is resumed
  - Is an uncommon cause of exercise-induced pain in the leg or foot
- Caused by an increase in the tissue pressure in the compartment resulting in compromise of tissue perfusion:
  - Limited or decreased volume of the compartment because of tight thickened fascia
  - Increased compartment content from muscle hypertrophy

Complement cascade

Why is knowledge of the complement cascade is of surgical importance?

- It is an important mechanism for control of infection
- It is important in the clotting cascade
- It can play a part in glomerulonephritis, which may cause renal failure requiring transplantation
- It is important in C1 esterase inhibitor deficiency

How does complement control infection?

- It is involved in bacterial killing
- It promotes phagocytosis and chemotaxis of leukocytes
- It promotes lymphocyte binding of antigens
- It is a mediator of inflammation through mast cell degranulation and chemotaxis

What is the essential difference between the classical and the alternate pathways of complement?

The classical pathway requires immunoglobulins to initiate it: the alternate pathway is independent of immunoglobulins for activation.

The classical pathway	The alternate pathway
• IgG or IgM molecules fix to a cell membrane • C1q binds to their long chains and then to C1r and C1s • The whole activates C4 and C2. C2,4 cleaves C3 into its components • C3a is chemotactic and anaphylactic. C3b is an opsonin and also acts with C2,4 to cleave C5 • C5a is chemotactic and anaphylactic. C5b binds with C6, C7, C8 and C9 to form the membrane attack complex	• The alternate pathway does not need activation by immunoglobulin • C3 is activated directly by endotoxins, viruses, bacteria, fungi and other particles

◼ Consent to operation

In the UK, the criteria for consent fall into three categories: the age, the physical state and the mental state of the patient.

What factors in terms of consent relate to the age of the patient?

- Any patient over 18 years can give consent for operation on themselves provided that his or her physical and mental state permits this
- When a patient under 16 years
  - He or she is a minor
  - His or her consent may be sought
  - The parents' consent is always sought
  - He or she can give consent to treatment without the parents' knowledge (the Gillick case) but this is still contentious
  - He or she cannot give consent to take part in medical research
- When a patient is aged 16 and 17 years
  - He or she can give consent to treatment
  - The parents' consent is usually sought
  - He or she cannot give consent to take part in medical research

If parents are considered to be acting against the interests of a child in terms of current medical practice, the senior surgeon treating the child can apply for the child to be made a ward of court.

What factors relate to the physical state of the patient?

- Doctors have a common law duty of care
- A "consent" form should be signed by the surgeon certifying that the patient is physically unable to make a decision on consent but that it is the surgeon's judgement that the treatment is essential
- When a patient cannot give consent because of unconsciousness the above applies provided that the patient before unconsciousness has not indicated that he or she refuses an operation
- A patient's next of kin cannot give or withhold consent, though of course their views should be sought

What factors relate to the mental state of the patient?

- Patients who have a mental disorder that is severe enough to warrant detention can be treated only for their psychiatric condition: they cannot be treated for a physical condition without their consent
- Patients with some psychiatric diseases can refuse treatment even when this would be lifesaving: intervention is not permitted
- Patients who are educationally challenged are treated as adults if they are over 16 years. Consent must be obtained. In terms of sterilisation and abortion, a court's decision is usually essential
- Any adult can refuse any investigation or treatment if they can understand the consequences of the refusal

■ Coroner I: referral

Under what circumstances must a death be referred to HM Coroner?

A death should be referred to the Coroner if:

- The cause of death is unknown
  - The cause of death really must be unknown – the Coroner must never be made to be the bogey man who forces a post-mortem examination despite reluctant relatives by removing the necessity for their consent
- The deceased was not seen by the certifying doctor after death and within the 14 days before death (the certifying doctor is the one who signs the death certificate, not the one who confirms that death has occurred)
- The death was violent or unnatural or there are suspicious circumstances
  - This section includes deaths that might be construed to have resulted as a consequence of surgery or to have been contributed to by surgery (or, of course, any of the other medical specialities). There is no statute of limitations – even if a patient survives for over a year, if the death can be linked materially to surgery it must be reported
- The death may be due to an accident (whenever it occurred)
  - Surgery might be construed as an accident: many surgical cases that appear before HMC are returned as accidental death (used to be called *death by misadventure*)

- The death may be due to self-neglect or neglect by others
  - Nursing staff perhaps, or intensive therapy unit (ITU) staff, or surgeons
- The death may be due to an industrial disease or may be directly related to the deceased's employment
  - In any case but especially if there is a pension involved. Can be tricky: a fall at work leading to death might or might not be related to the deceased's employment, depending on the circumstances
- The death may be due to an abortion
- The death occurred during an operation or before recovery from the effects of anaesthesia
- The death may be a suicide
  - Drug-related deaths are not always considered suicide: to die is not the first or second intention of most drug-takers
- The death occurred during or shortly after detention in police or prison custody
  - Or even ages afterwards if the police can be shown to have contributed materially to the death

■ Coroner II: verdicts

List some of the possible verdicts by a Coroner.

- Death from natural causes
- Death by accident ("misadventure" in the old terminology)
- Death from suicide
- Death aggravated by lack of care or self-neglect
- Death as a result of attempted or self-induced abortion
- Stillbirth
- Death from want of attention at birth
- Death from drug dependence
- Death from non-dependent abuse of drugs
- Death from industrial disease
- Death by homicide
- Unlawful killing (HMC will not give a verdict of murder or manslaughter)
- Lawful killing (by the police, armed forces or others of necessity)
- Death by natural disaster
- Open verdict (i.e. no verdict)
- Other, including treasure trove

■ Culture media

What are the two main types of culture medium in daily use?
- Solid media
- Liquid media

What are the advantages of each?
- Solid media permit isolation of separate colonies when there is a mixed growth
- Liquid media permit growth of some sensitive organisms using enrichment broths – used for blood cultures as there would be expected to be few organisms in the blood

What are the main types of solid media in daily use?
- Nutrient agar
- Blood agar
- MacConkey's agar

At operation, if pus is found that has a particularly foul smell, what should you suspect? What would you do to confirm this?

Infection by an anaerobic organism. Take a sample of pus directly to the microbiology laboratory for culture without delay. A capped syringe is preferable to a swab as this preserves the anaerobic conditions.

What are the main types of selective media, and for what do they select?

Media	Composition	Organisms
● MacConkey agar	Contains bile	Coliforms and other enterobacteria
● Salt agar	Contains NaCl	*Staphylococcus aureus*
● Lowenstein–Jensen medium	Contains malachite green, egg yolk and mineral salts	*Mycobacterium* spp.
● Antibiotic-containing media	Various antibiotics	*Neisseria gonorrhoeae*

■ Cushing's disease and syndrome

What is the essential biochemical abnormality in Cushing's disease and Cushing's syndrome?

- Hypercortisolaemia
- Harvey Williams Cushing (1896–1937), a neurosurgeon in Boston, Massachusetts published his widely recognised paper in 1932, though had published before that on the same subject in 1917

What is the difference between the disease and the syndrome?

- *Cushing's disease* is an abnormality of the pituitary gland, almost always an adenoma
- *Cushing's syndrome* is the recognised collection of symptoms and signs that result from hypercortisolaemia from any cause. Rarely the syndrome may be caused by Cushing's disease from pituitary adenoma
- A patient is diagnosed initially as having Cushing's syndrome. After investigations, he or she is found to have Cushing's disease or one of the other causes of the syndrome

What are the external features of a patient with severe Cushing's syndrome?

- Head and neck
  - Moon face from oedema and fat deposition from cortisol and aldosterone effects

- Acne from testosterone-like effects of cortisol
- Male pattern baldness
- Hirsutes in women
- Chest and trunk
  - Buffalo hump from change in adipose tissue distribution
  - Central obesity
  - Pendulous abdomen from loss of smooth muscle tone and accumulation of adipose tissue
  - Purple striae from thinning of skin
  - Ecchymoses from capillary fragility
  - Carbuncles, furuncles from diabetogenic effects
- Limbs
  - Muscle wasting from cortisol effect
  - Ecchymoses and petechiae

What are the internal features of a patient with severe Cushing's syndrome?

- Amenorrhoea from suppression of ovarian hormone secretion
- Changes of diabetes mellitus
- Bone changes, principally osteoporosis leading to compression fracture

What are the causes of Cushing's syndrome?

- iatrogenic: administration of steroids (common) and adrenocorticotropic hormone (ACTH) (rare)
- Patient administered steroids
- Adrenal adenoma and carcinoma

- Pituitary adenoma
- Ectopic secretion of an ACTH-like substance such as from:
  - Oat cell carcinoma
  - Carcinoid tumour
  - Islet cell tumour of pancreas

■ Cyst formation

What is a cyst?

An abnormal fluid-filled space characteristically lined by epithelial cells.

(Some spaces are called *cysts* when there is no epithelial lining and the contents are necrotic debris rather than simply fluid, such as an amoebic cyst in the liver. These will be included here.)

What pathological processes (such as inflammation, accumulation, degeneration) lead to the formation of a cyst?

- Congenital or developmental
  - Thyroglossal cyst
  - Branchial cyst
  - Biliary cyst
  - Pancreatic cyst
  - Lymphatic cyst as cystic hygroma
  - Some renal cysts
  - Some cysts of the CNS
  - Inclusion dermoid cyst
- Inflammation
  - Infective
    - Related to specific organisms
      - Amoebiasis
      - Cysticercosis
      - Hydatid disease

- ◆ Caused by obstruction
  - ▲ Some renal cysts
  - ▲ Spermatocele
  - ▲ Meibomian cyst
  - ▲ Epididymal cyst
  - ▲ Hydrosalpinx
  - ▲ True pancreatic cysts in chronic pancreatitis
- Degeneration (may be inflammatory or ischaemic)
  - ■ Bone cysts in osteoarthritis
  - ■ Cystic change in leiomyoma
  - ■ Cerebral cysts after infarction
- Implantation
  - ■ Epidermal cyst, dermal cyst
- Hyperplasia
  - ■ Breast and endometrial cysts
- Neoplasia
  - ■ Cystic neoplasms of the ovary
    - ◆ Benign cystic teratoma (dermoid cyst)
    - ◆ Serous, mucinous cystadenoma
    - ◆ Serous, mucinous cystadenocarcinoma
  - ■ Cystic neoplasms of the pancreas

What is the type of cyst commonly found on the scalp?

In most cases they are pilar cysts (also called *trichilemmal cysts*). Only about 10% are epidermal cysts, which are much commoner elsewhere in the skin. Sebaceous cysts (cysts formed from sebaceous glands or ducts) are very rare.

■ Diabetes mellitus

Why is diabetes mellitus of surgical as well as medical importance?

- Arterial disease
  - Atheroma
  - Arteriolosclerosis
  - Embolism
  - Aneurysm
- Renal damage requiring renal transplantation
  - Glomerulosclerosis: nodular (Kimmelsteil–Wilson) and diffuse
  - Tubular damage: ascending infection
  - Papillary necrosis: microangiopathy and ascending infection
  - Pyelonephritis from ascending infection
  - Renal artery stenosis from atheroma: atheroma virtually never affects the renal arteries themselves (as opposed to atheroma of the origins of the renal arteries, which is considered to be aortic disease) except in diabetes mellitus
  - Hypertensive damage to the kidneys as a consequence of diabetes mellitus
- Skin disease
  - Carbuncles and furuncles
  - Necrobiosis lipoidica diabeticorum
  - Wound healing
    - Infection
    - Denervation injury with anaesthesia

- General anaesthetic complications
- Eye disease
  - Cataracts
  - Proliferative retinopathy
  - Infections
- Bone and joint diseases
  - Septic arthritis
  - Osteomyelitis
- Systemic disturbance
  - Predisposition to
    - Metabolic crises
    - Septicaemia
    - Immune deficiency

■ Disseminated intravascular coagulopathy

Why is knowledge of disseminated intravascular coagulopathy (DIC) surgically important?

- Patients may present with DIC as a complication of a surgically treatable condition
- Patients with massive trauma may develop DIC and its subsequent complications
- Infections may cause DIC and complicate recovery from surgery
- Surgical intervention may cause DIC

How are the causes of DIC classified?

- Neoplastic
  - Carcinoma of the prostate, pancreas, bronchus, ovary: especially mucin-secreting tumours
- Massive tissue injury
  - Extensive surgical procedures
  - Burns
  - Major trauma
  - Fat embolus
- Infections
  - Viral
    - Haemorrhagic viral fevers
  - Bacterial
    - Meningococcal septicaemia
    - Gram-negative septicaemia

- Fungal
  - Aspergillosis
  - Systemic candidiasis
- Protozoal
  - Malaria
- Vascular and perfusion disorders
  - Vasculitis
    - Polyarteritis nodosa (PAN)
    - Systemic lupus erythematosus (SLE)
  - Aneurysm
  - Prosthetic grafts
  - Coarctation of the aorta
  - Adult respiratory distress syndrome (ARDS)
  - Myocardial infarction
- Haematological disorders
  - Leukaemias
  - Sickle cell disease
  - Intravascular haemolysis
- Others
  - Acute pancreatitis
  - Amniotic fluid embolism
  - Hypothermia

How is the clinical diagnosis of DIC confirmed?

- Low platelet count
- Low plasma fibrinogen
- Increased prothrombin time (PT), activated prothrombin time (APTT)
- Fibrin degradation products in urine and serum
- Haemolysis and fragmented red cells (schistocytes)

■ Diverticula

What is a diverticulum?
An abnormal outpouching of a hollow viscus into the surrounding tissues.

How are diverticula classified?
- Congenital and acquired
- True and false
- Pulsion and traction

What do true and false refer to?
- True diverticula have all of the components of the viscus wall
- False diverticula have only part of the wall represented

Is there any relation between these and congenital and acquired diverticula?
- True diverticula tend to be congenital and vice versa
- False diverticula tend to be acquired and vice versa

Give some examples of congenital diverticula
- Meckel's diverticulum
  - In the ileum 2 feet from the ileocaecal valve, 2 inches long, in 2% of the population
  - Always solitary
- Duodenal diverticula, which are usually multiple

Give some examples of false diverticula

- Sigmoid colon diverticulum
- Pharyngeal diverticulum through Killian's dehiscence between thyropharyngeus and cricopharyngeus muscles, the two components of the inferior pharyngeal constrictor

What are the complications of diverticula?

- Inflammation with or without infection
- Haemorrhage
- Perforation
- Blind loop syndrome causing vitamin deficiencies secondary to bacterial overgrowth
- Metaplasia, as in a bladder diverticulum from transitional epithelium to squamous
- Malignant change, as in bladder diverticula (but no increase in malignant potential in large bowel diverticula)
- Meckel's diverticulum
  - Meckel's diverticulitis
  - Ectopic gastric mucosa around the mouth, causing peptic ulceration of the ileum opposite the diverticulum
  - Intussusception
  - Patent vitellointestinal duct
  - Volvulus
  - Perforation

■ Dysplasia

What is the definition of dysplasia?

- Dysplasia in relation to neoplasia (the commonest use of the term)
  - A degree of failure of maturation of a tissue associated with a tendency to aneuploidy and pleomorphism but without the capacity of invasive spread. Severe dysplasia and carcinoma in situ may be considered synonymous; the tissue has all of the characteristics of malignancy but has not demonstrated stromal invasion.
  - Reference to invasion of basement membranes can lead to difficulties. There is good evidence that well-differentiated invasive neoplasms make basement membrane material around the islands of cells, and so undoubtedly invasive carcinoma can be shown to be surrounded by basement membrane.
- Dysplasia in relation to the abnormal formation of an organ or tissue (occasionally used for some specific lesions)
  - An abnormality of development of tissue in which fibrous or other non-specialised tissue is present instead of the expected specialised tissue. Examples include fibrous dysplasia of bone, in which there is fibrous tissue where bone might be expected.

At what sites is dysplasia relatively common?

- Cervix, now regarded as neoplasia and called cervical intraepithelial neoplasia (CIN)
- Bronchus, in relation to smoking

- Oesophagus, in relation to candidiasis (squamous dysplasia) and Barrett's change (glandular dysplasia)
- Stomach, in relation to *Helicobacter pylori* infection, usually on a background of intestinal metaplasia
- Large bowel, involved by ulcerative colitis

What are the causes of dysplasia?
- Smoking
- Viral infection, such as with human papilloma virus (HPV) types 16 and 18
- Specific types of chronic inflammation such as ulcerative colitis
- Non-specific types of chronic inflammation such as cystitis leading to bladder carcinoma
- Alcohol and other dietary constituents in relation to the larynx and stomach

What is the risk that an area of epithelial dysplasia will develop into invasive neoplasia?
Very variable. In the cervix, the chance of CIN 3 being associated with invasive cervical carcinoma is relatively high. In the stomach, the chance of gastric dysplasia being involved with gastric carcinoma is also relatively high. Dysplasia (actually intraepithelial neoplasia) in the vulva has only a 4% chance of invasive malignancy.

What are the histological features of dysplasia?
- Multilayering of a columnar of cuboidal epithelium
- Mitotic figures

- Increased numbers of normal mitoses
- Presence of abnormal mitoses, such as
  - Sunburst mitoses (which look like prophase mitoses but with too many chromosomes)
  - Tripolar mitoses (with three centromeres pulling three ways)
  - Bizarre mitoses (with completely abnormal forms)
- Pleomorphism
- Hyperchromatism
- Loss of cell–cell cohesion, resulting in shedding
- *No* invasion into the underlying connective tissue

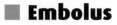

■ Embolus

Define *embolus.*

An embolus is an abnormal mass of undissolved material that is carried in the bloodstream from one place to another.

Some definitions include a requirement for the embolus to impact. This usually occurs but is not essential to the definition – an amniotic fluid embolus has no capacity to impact.

What is an embolus composed of?

About 95% of all emboli are thrombi or mixtures of thrombus and clot. Others include:

- Tumour cells, characteristically from
  - Malignant tumours especially carcinomas, either singly or in small groups
- Fat, characteristically from
  - Fractured long bones in adults but occasionally in patients with severe burns or extensive soft tissue injuries and in patients having orthopaedic procedures involving pressure on bone marrow such as intramedullary nailing
- Bone marrow, characteristically from
  - Fractured long bones in children
- Atheromatous material, characteristically from
  - Rupture of aortic plaques with emboli to mesenteric vessels

- Air, characteristically from
  - Cannulae, opened neck veins from trauma or head-and-neck surgery, dialysis procedures, and fallopian tube or peritoneal insufflation
- Nitrogen, characteristically in
  - Caisson disease (not Caisson's disease: a caisson is the box or compression chamber used for building bridges). At high pressures air dissolves in plasma and connective tissues. The oxygen from the air forced into solution is used by cells for respiration, leaving behind nitrogen and inert gases to form bubbles in the spinal cord, bones, joints, brain and elsewhere
- Amniotic fluid, characteristically in
  - Labour, leading to disseminated intravascular coagulopathy
- Infective agents, such as parasites like schistosomes and bacteria in infective endocarditis with embolisation
- Diatoms and other organisms, characteristically from
  - Rivers and the sea, transported from the lungs to the bone marrow in people who drown, evidence that death was due to inhalation of water and not laryngeal spasm and suffocation as a result of being immersed
- Foreign material, such as plastic tubing from broken cannulae, talc in drug addicts

■ Epistaxis

What is epistaxis?
Acute haemorrhage from the nostril, nasal cavity or nasopharynx.

How is epistaxis classified?
By whether the primary bleeding site is anterior or posterior:
- Most commonly anterior
  - The anterior aspect of the septum
  - Commonly from Kiesselbach's plexus, a network of veins just superior to the posterior end of the vestibule (also called Little's area)
  - Occasionally anterior to the inferior turbinate
- Much less commonly posterior
  - The posterior aspect of the nasal cavity usually below the posterior half of the inferior turbinate or roof of the nasal cavity
  - The nasopharynx

What causes epistaxis?
Most cases are idiopathic. Hypertension is rarely a direct cause though it might contribute. Causes include:
- Local trauma by nose picking
- Foreign bodies
- Inflammation
  - Nasal or sinus infections
  - Allergy, seasonal rhinitis, atrophic rhinitis

- Desiccation from prolonged inhalation of dry air
  - Disturbance of normal nasal airflow, as from a deviated nasal septum, may contribute
- Patients with a bleeding tendency
  - Thrombocytopaenia
  - Disseminated intravascular coagulopathy
  - Leukaemias and lymphomas
  - Congenital bleeding diatheses: haemophilia, von Willebrand's disease
  - Chronic liver disease
- Barotrauma
- Cocaine use
- Iatrogenic
  - Nasogastric and nasotracheal intubation
  - Heparin and warfarin
  - Aspirin and other non-steroidal anti-inflammatory agents
  - Cytotoxic drugs
- Rarer causes
  - Hereditary haemorrhagic telangiectasia
  - Arteriovenous malformations
  - Neoplasia
  - Endometriosis

How can epistaxis be controlled?

In most cases:
- Pinch nostrils, lean forward
- Cautery with silver nitrate
- Nasal pack

In severe cases:

- Endoscopic cautery
- Laser cautery
- Postnasal packing
- Embolisation
- Arterial ligation
  - Anterior ethmoidal artery ligation
  - Maxillary artery ligation
  - External carotid artery ligation in extremis

■ Exotoxins and endotoxins

Define exotoxin and endotoxin.

An exotoxin is an immunogenic protein secreted from a living organism that is heat labile and has a specific molecular target.

Exotoxins may act as:

- Enzymes: *Vibrio cholerae* toxin, *Corynaebacterium diphtheriae* toxin
- Neurotoxins: tetanospasmin from *Clostridium tetani*, *Clostridium botulinum* toxin
- Disrupters of the plasma membranes of target cells: *Clostridium perfringens* toxin, *Staphylococcus aureus* toxin, *Streptococcus pyogenes* toxin

An endotoxin is a lipopolysaccharide derived from the cell wall of an organism that is not usually immunogenic, is heat stable, and has a non-specific, wide-ranging effects on many molecular targets.

Endotoxins result in:

- Cytokine formation
- Fibrin degradation
- Activation of the clotting cascade
- Kinin formation
- Nitric oxide formation
- Prostaglandin formation
- Complement activation
- Platelet-activating factor formation
- Leucotriene formation

What diseases are caused by toxins?

- Exotoxins
  - Cholera: profuse watery diarrhoea and no ulceration of the bowel
  - Diphtheria: only strains that are infected by a bacteriophage produce toxin
  - Gas gangrene from *Clostridium perfringens* and other clostridia
  - Food poisoning with onset after only a few hours of ingestion of the infected food
  - Botulism and tetanus from *Clostridium botulinum* and *tetani*
- Endotoxins
  - Shock
  - Disseminated intravascular coagulopathy
  - Hypotension
  - Pyrexia
  - Organ failure

First and second intention wound healing

What does healing by first and second intention mean?

- First intention healing refers to clean, surgical wounds without tissue loss that heal with minimal fibrosis
- Second intention healing refers to wounds that have tissue loss or are intentionally left open, and so develop granulation tissue to fill the gap and heal by fibrosis

What events take place in the epidermis during healing?

- Clot forms at the injury site
- Epithelial cells migrate from the wound edges by amoeboid movement to cover the clot
- This migration depends on the interaction of keratinocytes with fibronectin
- Integrins on keratinocytes bind to fibronectin
- Integrins that bind to fibronectin are not present on keratinocytes in the undamaged skin
- Proliferation of keratinocytes contributes to the ability to cover the wound

What events take place in the dermis during healing?

- Infiltration of polymorphs and macrophages to remove debris
- Fibroblast activity to restore tensile strength
- Revascularisation
- Myofibroblast contraction

What growth factors are involved in wound healing?

- Platelet-derived and other growth factors
  - Synthesised by macrophages, endothelial cells, smooth muscle cells which attract mesenchymal cells into the wound
  - Act as mitogens for these cells
- Epidermal growth factor (EGF), found in:
  - Saliva
  - Tears
  - Duodenal secretions (EGF used to be called urogastrone)
  - Platelet α-granules which accelerate epidermal and dermal regeneration
- Transforming growth factor β, which acts:
  - As a mitogen
  - As a chemoattractant
- Cytokines, which include:
  - Lymphokines
  - Monocytokines
  - Interleukins

■ Food poisoning

In terms of time of onset after ingestion of infected food, how is food poisoning divided into three?

- Early onset after 3–5 hours
- Onset after 8–15 hours
- Onset after 24 hours

What are the causes of early onset food poisoning?

Preformed exotoxins in the food from infection by *Staphylococcus aureus* or *Bacillus cereus*.

What are the causes of food poisoning about 8–15 hours after ingestion?

Exotoxins from organisms such as *Clostridium perfringens*.

What are the causes of food poisoning 24 hours after ingestion?

Endotoxins from organisms such as *Campylobacter jejuni* and *Shigella sonnei*.

What toxins are produced by *Escherichia coli*?

- Enteropathogenic
- Enterotoxigenic
- Enteroinvasive
- Enterohaemorrhagic (*Escherichia coli* 0157)

■ Formalin and its effects on tissues

Why is formaldehyde a good fixative?

- Its cost
  - It is very cheap and diluted further after purchase
- Its versatility
  - Formalin fixes all tissues well. When electron microscopy is required glutaraldehyde fixation is better, but tissues can be post-fixed in glutaraldehyde after formalin fixation. All of the immunostains in common use work on formalin-fixed tissues
- Its preservative properties
  - Tissue components are fixed in place by cross-linkages with formalin so preserving relations
  - Antigenicity is preserved to a great extent, permitting immunohistochemical staining of cell constituents and of collagen, laminin and other extracellular materials
  - The water content prevents dehydration
  - Formalin is bactericidal and fungicidal, and so prevents denaturation by infection
- Its compatibility with haematoxylin and eosin staining
  - Haematoxylin and eosin (H&E) is universal: all countries in the world use it as standard, and formalin fixation contributes to its uniformity, and so acceptability

What are the problems with fixation using formalin?

- Toxicity
  - Formalin is severely irritant as a solution and as a vapour. Histopathologists can develop skin rashes and anosmia

- Misuse
  - The best volume ratio of formalin is more than 100 times the volume of formalin to the volume of the tissue to be fixed. Tissues crammed into pots with only a few millilitres of formalin cannot fix and will decay; as a consequence, the pressure in the specimen container will increase and when opened formalin will spray into the pathologist's eyes

■ Fracture healing

Starting at the moment of fracture, what are the stages of healing of the fracture of a long bone?

- Haematoma formation
  - Size limited by the elastic periosteum when this is intact and by arterial spasm
- Inflammatory phase
  - Vascular dilatation, exudate, polymorph infiltration
- Demolition phase
  - Macrophages digest clot, fibrin and debris; macrophages and osteoclasts remove dead bone fragments
- Organisation
  - Granulation tissue formation with ingrowth of capillary loops from below the periosteum and from the fractured bone ends
- Early callus formation
  - Osteoid is laid down in a haphazard arrangement of fibrils which mineralise to form woven bone. Cartilage may also be formed especially when there is movement at the fracture site
- Late callus formation
  - Woven bone is absorbed by osteoclasts and osteoblasts, which lay down lamellar bone with Haversian systems
- Remodelling
  - The normal shape of the bone is remodelled over many months and the marrow cavity reforms

What abnormalities of fracture healing can occur?

- Fibrous union
  - When movement of the fracture site is free the bone ends unite by fibrous tissue. When there is excessive movement differentiation into synovial cells may result with the formation of a pseudo-arthrosis
- Non-union
  - When there is interposition of soft parts, usually muscle or fascia. Occasionally, the interposition of a foreign body may cause non-union
- Delayed union because of
  - Sepsis, especially in comminuted or compound fractures
  - Foreign body
  - Movement of the fracture site
  - Ischaemia, especially in fracture of the neck of the femur, shaft of tibia and scaphoid
- Malunion
  - With consequent osteoarthritis

■ Free radicals

What is a free radical?

An atom or molecule that has an unpaired electron in its outer orbit. They are highly reactive and can create further free radicals by their effects on cell components.

Give some examples of free radicals.

H·, OH·, COO·, OOH·, C·

What causes free radicals to form?

- Radiation energy absorbed by cell constituents
- Drugs and chemicals such as paraquat and carbon tetrachloride
- Oxygen in toxic concentrations and sometimes in physiological concentrations
- Lysosomal reactions in the killing of bacteria

What are the molecular effects of free radicals?

- Protein damage
- DNA damage
- Lipid peroxidation leading to loss of calcium channel control
- Degradation of glycosaminoglycans in connective tissues

In what diseases are free radicals considered to be important?

- Inflammation
- Chemical and drug injuries
- Oxygen toxicity
- Atheroma
- Radiation damage
- Ageing – ceroid and lipofuscin formation
- Carcinogenesis

■ Frozen section diagnosis

What are the indications for frozen section?

- As an intra-operative diagnostic tool in very limited circumstances
- The patient's immediate management must be dependent on the result of the frozen section (FS) examination
- The question asked must be within the capacity of a FS examination to answer it:
  - FS is useful in determining whether a lesion is benign or malignant, such as in the differential diagnosis of a frozen pelvis caused by cervical carcinoma or endometriosis
  - FS is useless in trying to distinguish lymphoma from a reactive condition causing lymph node enlargement (and may actually be contraindicated if the specimen is the only one that will be available on which a definitive diagnosis is to be made)
- Examination of excision margins to know whether a carcinoma has been excised completely, especially when the least amount of excision may be preferable as in laryngectomy and glossectomy
- Tissue identification: to establish that a parathyroid gland is not a lymph node or a protrusion of thyroid
- As a procedure unrelated directly to the operative surgery, such as for enzyme studies on muscle biopsies and polymerase chain reaction (PCR) on cervical biopsies. Most immunostains nowadays work well on fixed tissues processed to paraffin wax blocks and so FS is becoming unnecessary.

What are the limitations of a FS examination that a surgeon must be aware of?

- The process is destructive: a small specimen can be destroyed by freezing because of ice-crystal artefact
- There will be false-negatives and false-positives, more frequently than in routine histopathological practice
- There will be sampling problems, important in follicular thyroid nodules and some ovarian carcinomas
- The diagnosis will usually be simplified – cancer or not cancer – rather than the fine-tuned diagnosis that is possible from properly processed tissues
- The diagnosis might be misleading; distortion of the tissues on FS can make tuberculosis look like carcinoma or sarcoma
- It is expensive; FS disrupts the routine working of the laboratory considerably

■ Fungi

How do fungi differ from bacteria?
- Fungi are generally larger
- Fungal cells have nuclei with multiple chromosomes and cytoplasm containing mitochondria and ribosomes
- Many fungi can reproduce sexually

How are fungi classified?
- Yeasts
- Filamentous fungi
- Dimorphic fungi

How do fungi cause disease?
- By infection
  - Superficial as in candidal infection of mucosal surfaces and dermatophytes causing nail infections
  - Subcutaneous after implantation of fungus as in tropical mycoses
  - Systemic when there is widespread haematogenous dissemination especially if there is an indwelling catheter
- By toxin production
  - Such as aflatoxin from *Aspergillus flavus* and ergot from *Claviceps purpurea*
- By hypersensitivity reactions
  - Such as against *Aspergillus*, which can provoke a type I or III reaction

Which patients are prone to fungal infections?

- Patients with diabetes
- Immunocompromised patients
  - With cancer, especially leukaemia and lymphoma
  - With AIDS
  - Receiving wide-spectrum antibiotics, immunosuppressive drugs, cytotoxic drugs with deficient T-cell function leading to chronic mucocutaneous candidosis
- Premature infants
- Patients with an indwelling central venous pressure (CVP) line

▪ Gastric cancer

What are the principal types of gastric cancer?

Adenocarcinoma, leiomyosarcoma, gastrointestinal stromal tumour and gastric lymphoma.

What are the two types of adenocarcinoma of the stomach?

- Intestinal type
  - Commoner than diffuse type
  - Forms polypoid masses
  - Has gland formation with intraglandular mucin
  - Predominates in countries with a high incidence of gastric cancer
  - Ulcerates
  - Has a slightly better prognosis than the diffuse type
- Diffuse type
  - Spreads through the wall without forming a polypoid mass – "leatherbottle stomach" (linitis plastica is a misnomer: it is neither inflammatory nor plastic)
  - Has no gland formation and instead forms signet-ring cells with intracellular mucin

What are the risk factors for gastric adenocarcinoma?

- Diet
  - Excessive salt intake: sodium chloride and sodium nitrite (used in Japanese cooking)
  - Excessive consumption of smoked or pickled foods

- Excessive consumption of alcohol, especially undiluted spirits
- Possibly consumption of asbestos as a contaminant of talc used to polish rice and of coal seams
  - Coal miners in Utah are eight times more likely to develop adenocarcinoma than people in non-mining areas of the USA
- Low intake of milk, fresh fruit and vegetables
  - β-carotene and vitamin C decrease the risk of gastric cancer
  - Frozen foods decrease the risk, possibly related to the above
- *Helicobacter pylori* infection
- Long-standing reflux
- Chronic gastritis, especially with intestinal metaplasia, with or without ulceration
- Pernicious anaemia and other types of atrophic gastritis
- Familial adenomatous polyposis (FAP) and gastric polyps unrelated to FAP
- Family history with a first-degree relative affected
- Smoking
- Ethnic origin: commoner in Japan, Chile and Iceland; commoner in American Blacks, Asians and Hispanics than American Whites
- Sex: men are three times more likely to be affected than women
- Age: over 50 years the risk climbs – fewer than 10% of cases occur in people under 50 years

- Almost certainly *not* blood group: gastric adenocarcinoma is commonest in people with blood group B (not A as given in many books) as it is the commonest group in Japan

How has gastric adenocarcinoma changed in recent times?

- In the world, one-third as common now as it was 50 years ago
- Most tumours were in the pyloric area but now the commonest site is in the cardia
- Five-year survival rates have doubled but are still only 12%
- Screening programmes have reduced the prevalence of the intestinal type of gastric adenocarcinoma; the diffuse or signet-ring type has not been affected

■ Genetics: surgical aspects

Why should a surgeon know something about genes and genetics?

- Screening
  - Some diseases amenable to surgery can be screened for the genetic susceptability, such as familial adenomatous polyposis, breast carcinoma and some forms of thyroid carcinoma
- Early diagnosis
  - Early detection of tumours that have a surgical cure or palliation might be possible such as by demonstration of microsatellite instability in some surgically amenable lung cancers and *k-ras* growth promoter activity in colorectal adenomas and small cell carcinomas
- Genetic staging
  - Staging by the molecular detection of tumour mRNA in lymph nodes affected by metastases when histological examination is negative. The significance of these genetically detectable micrometastases is not known
- Prognostic markers
  - Overexpression of *c-erb*B-2 in about 25% of breast carcinomas is associated with tumour relapse after surgery
  - Microsatellite instability appears to have a survival advantage in colorectal carcinoma
  - *k-ras* expression is associated with a decreased survival in patients with colorectal carcinoma

- Pharmacogenetics as therapy
  - Transfection of tumours with genes that produce proteins which metabolise a pro-cytotoxic to a cytotoxic drug; this can reduce the plasma concentrations of the prodrug needed to non-toxic levels with efficient treatment of hepatic metastases of colorectal carcinoma
  - Immunotherapy with cytokine-producing genes that make, for example, interleukins which can limit the growth of hepatic metastases of colorectal carcinoma
  - Genes for p53 in its unmutated, active form can be introduced into lung carcinomas with advantageous therapeutic effects
- Identification of virulence factors and vascular growth factors
  - Vascular endothelial growth factor can be used for critical limb ischaemia
  - Genetic variations can lead to different susceptibility to pancreatitis among patients with cystic fibrosis

■ Giant cells

What is a giant cell?

There is no agreed definition, but any cell that is more than 10 times the size of a lymphocyte would be considered to be a giant cell.

How are giant cells classified?

- Normal
  - Osteoclasts
  - Skeletal muscle cells
  - Syncytiotrophoblasts
  - Megakaryocytes
  - Oocytes and ova
- Abnormal
  - Macrophage and related giant cells present in disease
    - Foreign body (FB) multinucleate giant cells in FB reactions
    - Langhans' cells in TB, sarcoidosis, Crohn's disease
    - Touton giant cells in xanthoma, xanthelasma
  - Virus induced
    - Warthin–Finkeldey giant cells in measles (derived from lymphocytes)
    - Cytomegalovirus giant cells
    - Herpes-simplex-induced multinucleate giant cells
  - Tumour giant cells
    - Giant cell tumour of bone (osteoclastoma)
    - Reed Sternberg cells in Hodgkin's disease (which are modified B-lymphocytes)

- Bizarre epithelial giant cells in anaplastic carcinomas
- Bizarre glial giant cells in grade 4 astrocytoma
- Others
  - Adrenal cytomegaly (congenital and acquired)
  - Thyroid cytomegaly (dyshormonogenesis)

◼ Gout I: surgical relevance and derivation

Why is knowledge of gout of surgical as well as medical importance?
- Joint diseases
  - Differential diagnosis of septic arthritis
  - Crystal arthropathies of which gout is one (also calcium pyrophosphate arthropathy, "pseudogout")
  - Osteoarthritis as a consequence of gout
- Urinary tract calculi from urate deposition
- Gouty tophi might need cosmetic surgery
- Complications of treatment with cytotoxic agents and radiotherapy that cause massive cell death and therefore gout

Must a patient with gout have hyperuricaemia? Must a patient with hyperuricaemia develop gout?
No and no, though in fact usually yes in both cases.

What is uric acid derived from?
Purines (adenine, guanine) are metabolised differently from pyrimidines (uracil and thymine in DNA, uracil and cytosine in RNA). Only purines are involved in hyperuricaemia.

What is the difference between a nucleoside and a nucleotide?
A nucleoside is a purine or pyrimidine (a base) joined with a form of ribose, a sugar.

In RNA this is a ribonucleoSIDE, and in DNA a deoxyribonucleoSIDE.

Ribonucleosides and deoxyribonucleosides are usually linked to phosphate radicals, when they are known as nucleoTIDEs, for example, adenosine diphosphate (ADP) and adenosine triphosphate (ATP).

How are purines and pyrimidines metabolised?

Purines are degraded to hypoxanthine, which is then changed by xanthine oxidase to xanthine, then to uric acid which is excreted in urine (hence allopurinol, a xanthine oxidase inhibitor, can be useful in treatment).

Pyrimidines are unrelated to hyperuricaemia and gout. They are degraded into ammonium salts and urea (which is biochemically completely unrelated to uric acid).

■ Gout II: classification and complications

How is hyperuricaemia classified?

- Primary
  - Absolute or relative abnormality of xanthine–hypoxanthine handling
    - ♦ Deficiency of phosphoribosyl transferase means that xanthine and hypoxanthine cannot be recycled into purines and so must be excreted. The end point of their metabolism in human beings is uric acid
- Secondary
  - Increased purine breakdown with increased formation of uric acid
    - ♦ Increased cell turnover and apoptosis
      - ▲ Severe psoriasis
      - ▲ Malignant tumours such as leukaemia, myeloproliferative diseases, especially after chemotherapy
    - ♦ Decreased excretion of urate
      - ▲ Chronic renal failure, thiazide diuretics, other drugs

What are the complications of gout?

- Orthopaedic problems from osteoarthritis because of destructive joint disease
- Renal calculi from urate stones, and their complications
- Renal failure from massive deposition in the kidneys in patients treated with cytotoxic drugs or radiotherapy
- Radiological appearances that might be mistaken for neoplasia

■ Granulocytes

Classify polymorphonuclear leucocytes.

Polymorphs are classed as neutrophils, basophils and eosinophils:

- Neutrophils have
    - Polysegmented nuclei with four to five lobes (rising to six to seven lobes in patients with vitamin B_{12} or folate deficiency)
    - Clear cytoplasm and fine amphophilic granules that contain
        - Elastase
        - Protease
        - α-1-antitrypsin
        - Lysozyme
        - Lactoferrin
    - A role in acute inflammation and digestion of small particles such as bacteria
- Basophils have
    - Unlobated or bilobate nuclei
    - Basophilic granules (blue on routine stains) that contain
        - Histamine
        - Eosinophil chemotactic factor
        - Slow-releasing substance of anaphylaxis
    - Importance in allergic reactions and anaphylaxis
- Eosinophils have
    - Bilobed nuclei
    - Brightly eosinophilic granules that contain

- Major basic protein
- Eosinophil cationic protein
- Importance in reactions to parasites such as schistosomes and other metazoa, and also with neoplasms of the cervix and lung

Are basophils the circulating counterpart of mast cells?

No. Mast cells are capable of multiplication and live in the tissues for a considerable time: basophils are incapable of multiplication and have a short life only in the circulation.

The two cell lines may share a common bone-marrow precursor and do have cytoplasmic constituents in common, but it is no longer considered that tissue mast cells are derived directly from circulating basophils.

■ Gynaecology

Why should surgeons know about gynaecological problems?

- In the differential diagnosis of right and left iliac fossa pain
  - Mittelschmertz
  - Ruptured ectopic pregnancy
  - Salpingitis and perioophoritis
  - Torsion of ovarian cyst
  - Ovarian neoplasia
  - Endometriosis
  - Retrograde menstruation
- In the differential diagnosis of an abdominal mass
  - Pregnant uterus
  - Uterine fibroids
  - Hydrosalpinx
  - Ovarian neoplasia
  - Endometriosis
- Carcinoma of large bowel might involve the female genital organs, and so have implications for presenting features, diagnosis, operative management and prognosis
- Malignant ascites could be from ovarian carcinoma as well as gastric and colonic carcinoma and this must be considered in management

■ Haemolytic anaemia

How is haemolytic anaemia classified?

- Inherited
  - Red cell membrane abnormalities
    - Spherocytosis
    - Elliptocytosis (usually asymptomatic)
    - Abetalipoproteinaemia
  - Haemoglobin abnormalities
    - Sickle cell disease
    - Haemoglobinopathies such as HbC, HbD Punjab, HbE
    - Thalassaemia
  - Enzyme abnormalities
    - Glucose-6-phosphate dehydrogenase (G-6-PD) deficiency and favism
    - Pyruvate kinase deficiency
    - Glutathione synthetase deficiency
- Acquired
  - Immune
    - Autoimmune: cold agglutinins, drug-induced haemolysis
    - Isoimmune: ABO and Rh incompatibilities
  - Mechanical
    - Artificial heart valves
    - Microangiopathic haemolytic anaemia

How is haemolytic anaemia diagnosed?

- Low haemoglobin: normochromic normocytic anaemia, or an apparent macrocytic anaemia on a Coulter result because of reticulocytosis
- Raised reticulocyte count in peripheral blood
- Excess serum unconjugated bilirubin
- Absence in the urine of bilirubin
- Decreased serum haptoglobin concentration
- Increased serum methaemalbumin (methaemoglobin bound to albumin) concentration
- Increased red cell creatine concentration

◼ Hamartoma

What is the definition of a hamartoma?

A focal or multifocal malformation composed of a haphazard arrangement of different amounts of the tissues normally found at that site. This word derives from the Greek for error or sin. A choristoma is a tumour-like malformation composed of tissues *not* normally found at that site usually as a developmental tumour or tumour-like condition.

Why is knowledge of hamartomas surgically important?

It is important to be aware that a non-neoplastic mass can arise as a simple developmental error at different sites because of the potential for misdiagnosis as a neoplasm, with consequent overtreatment, morbidity and mortality.

In an uncomplicated hamartoma there is no tendency for the lesion to grow other than under the normal growth controls of the body. This does not mean that hamartomas are harmless.

How do hamartomas cause morbidity?

- Obstruction
- Pressure, which may be direct or indirect
- Infection
- Infarction
- Haemorrhage and iron-deficiency anaemia
- Fracture
- Mistaken diagnosis of malignancy
- Development of neoplasia

For example, when skeletal growth ceases at the age of 18 or 20 years, an osteochondroma of long bone stops growing. This occurs in most cases: neoplasia may rarely develop in the cartilage cap, and so the commonest complicating neoplasm is a chondrosarcoma.

Give some examples of hamartomas.

- Haemangioma and other vascular tumours that are not true neoplasms
- Peutz–Jeghers' polyp of bowel, juvenile polyp of large bowel
- Bronchial hamartoma
- Melanocytic naevi
- Neurofibromatosis as in von Recklinghausen's disease
- Bizarre neuroepithelial cells in tuberose sclerosis
- Overgrowth of developmental remnants may be considered hamartomatous if they represent a discrete tumour-like mass

Can a true neoplasm arise in a hamartoma?

- Chondrosarcoma arising in osteochondroma
- Neurofibrosarcoma in patients with von Recklinghausen's disease

Can a neoplasm be associated with hamartomas without arising in one?

- Fibroma of ovary in patients with Peutz–Jeghers' syndrome
- Malignant ovarian tumours arising in patients with Peutz–Jeghers' syndrome

■ Head injury

What are the indications for admission after head injury?

These include patients who:

- Have had loss of consciousness
- Have amnesia of more than 5 minutes back-duration
- Have abnormal neurological symptoms and signs
- Are confused or who have a depressed level of consciousness
- Are unwell from any reason
- Have complicating factors such as diabetes mellitus
- Have a reason for intracranial haemorrhage from their history
- Are found to have a skull fracture
- Might have a spinal injury
- Cannot be assessed
- Cannot be discharged into the care of an appropriate person

What are the principles and parts of the Glasgow Coma Score (GCS)?

The GCS assesses motor responses, verbal responses and eye-opening responses on a defined scale. Severe head injury is defined as a GCS of 8 or less. The GCS can be used dynamically as well as on the first encounter; a deterioration in a patient's condition of more than 3 points is an indication for immediate reassessment and a CT scan:

- Motor responses
  - Spontaneous: 6
  - Localised motor response to pain: 5

- Withdraws from pain in a non-specific manner: 4
- Abnormal flexion movements: 3
- Abnormal extension movements: 2
- No response: 1
- Verbal responses
  - Appropriate speech: 5
  - Confused speech: 4
  - Inappropriate single words: 3
  - Incomprehensible noises: 2
  - None: 1
- Eye-opening responses
  - Spontaneous: 4
  - Open as response to speech: 3
  - Open as response to pain: 2
  - No eye-opening: 1

■ *Helicobacter pylori*

What type of an organism is *Helicobacter pylori*?
- A Gram-negative spiral bacterium
- Discovered in 1893 in the gastric mucosa of dogs, then forgotten
- Identified in 1983 in the gastric mucosa of human beings
- Affects over half the world's population
- Infection begins in childhood
- Increases in prevalence with age
- Affects Blacks more than Whites

What diseases are known to be related to *Helicobacter pylori* infection?
- Gastritis
- Duodenal ulcer
- Gastric ulcer
- Gastric adenocarcinoma
- Gastric lymphoma
- Barrett's oesophagus probably

What tests are available for diagnosis?
- Serum antibody test
  - Identifies specific IgA or IgG
  - If present, indicate either current or past infection
  - Not always reliable
  - Cannot be used to see whether treatment has worked – antibodies take years to disappear after the infection is cured

- Gastric or duodenal mucosal biopsy
  - Enzyme tests for urease production
  - Histological examination
    - Haematoxylin and eosin (H&E)
    - Special stains for *Helicobacter pylori*
  - Culture
    - If bacteria grow (and they might not) sensitivity testing is possible
- Urease breath test
  - Radiolabelled urea (tagged with ^{14}C or ^{13}C) is broken down by urease
  - Labelled carbon dioxide that is released is collected and measured
  - Unmetabolised urea is excreted in urine
- Stool antigen test
  - Less expensive than the other tests
  - Results can be obtained in about 3 hours
  - Determines whether treatment has been successful

■ Hepatitis

What are the causes of acute hepatitis?
Hepatitis viruses, other viruses that affect the liver as part of a generalised infection, drugs and chemicals, and other causes.

Which are the specific hepatitis viruses?
- Hepatitis A virus
  - RNA virus
  - Picornavirus family
  - Faeco-oral route of transmission
- Hepatitis B virus
  - The only DNA hepatitis virus
  - Hepadnavirus family
  - Parenteral spread, sexual spread, spread from mother to fetus
- Hepatitis C virus
  - RNA virus
  - Flavivirus family
  - Parenteral and sexual spread
- Hepatitis D virus
  - RNA virusoid or delta agent, an incomplete virus
  - Parenteral and sexual spread
- Hepatitis E virus
  - RNA virus
  - Calcivirus family
  - Faeco-oral and possibly water-borne spread
- Hepatitis G virus
  - Similar to Hepatitis C virus

- RNA virus
- Parenteral and sexual spread

What viruses affect the liver as part of a generalised infection of other tissues?

- Herpes viruses
  - Epstein–Barr virus
  - Herpes simplex virus
  - Varicella-zoster virus
  - Cytomegalovirus (CMV)
- Flaviviruses
  - Yellow fever
  - Dengue
- Adenoviruses
- Enteroviruses
- Arenaviruses
  - Lassa fever virus
- Filoviruses
  - Marburg virus
  - Ebola virus

What other causes of acute hepatitis are there?

- Pregnancy
- Drugs
  - Dose dependent: ethanol, salicylates, paracetamol
  - Dose independent: isoniacid, phenytoin, amiodarone, halothane, statins
- Chemical toxic agents such as carbon tetrachloride and benzene

What are the complications of acute hepatitis?

- Fulminant hepatitis
- Chronic hepatitis
- Cirrhosis
- Hepatocellular carcinoma
- Hepatorenal syndrome
- Complications of liver failure
  - Coagulopathy
  - Encephalopathy
  - Electrolyte imbalance and oedema from hypoproteinuria
  - Inability to metabolise active substances such as aldosterone causing secondary hyperaldosteronism

■ Herniation

What is a hernia?

A protrusion of a viscus or tissue from the body compartment in which it normally resides into another body compartment. This may be complete (e.g. inguinal, femoral herniation) or partial (Richter's, sliding gastric).

What are the predisposing features to herniation?

- Increased pressure in the donor compartment
    - Increased abdominal pressure resulting in
        - Inguinal hernia
        - Femoral hernia: three times commoner in women than in men, but women have three times more inguinal hernia repairs than femoral
        - Obturator hernia
        - Diaphragmatic hernias
            - Morgagni
            - Bochdalek
            - Hiatus
    - Increased intracranial pressure resulting in
        - Prolapse of the cingulate gyrus under the falx cerebri
        - Mid-line shift of the pineal gland, pituitary gland
        - Prolapse of the brain through the tentorium and foramen magnum
- Congenital absence of normal tissue
    - Congenital diaphragmatic hernia with aplastic muscle and aplasia of the lung on the same side

- Weakness of tissues with normal pressure in the donor compartment
  - Incisional hernia
    - ◆ General factors such as nutrition, chronic airways limitation, immunodeficiency
    - ◆ Specific factors at the original operation such as
      - ▲ Poor technique
      - ▲ Haematoma
      - ▲ Infection

What are the complications of herniation?

- Obstruction of a hollow viscus
- Ischaemia and infarction
  - The small bowel in an inguinal hernia (incarceration and strangulation)
  - The limbic system in downward displacement through the tentorium cerebelli
  - The corpus callosum in herniation below the falx cerebri
- Pressure on structures normally present at the hernia site, such as
  - The midbrain
  - The medulla and upper spinal cord
- Pressure effects usually unrelated to ischaemia, such as
  - On the lungs in diaphragmatic hernia
- Cardiac arrhythmias associated with para-oesophageal hernia
- Rupture
- Reflux, such as of gastric contents

■ Histology and cytology

How are tissues sampled for histology?
- Biopsy by
  - Wide bore needle
  - Scrape or shave biopsy such as for basal cell carcinoma of skin
  - Biopsy forceps
  - Diathermy loop
  - Deep biopsy such as cone biopsy of cervix
- Excision by
  - Biopsy forceps (for a very small lesion)
  - Diathermy loop
  - Scalpel

And for cytology?
- *Exfoliative*: cervix, skin
- *Brushings*: bronchus, stomach
- *Fluid examination*: ascites, pleural effusion, lavage recovery
- *Fine needle aspiration*: thyroid, lymph nodes
- *Imprint onto a slide*: lymph nodes, spleen

What are the benefits of each?

	Histology	Cytology
Number of cells sampled	Large	Large
Field sampled	Small	Large
Field definition	Local	Large and poorly defined usually
Architecture	Assessable	Lost
Invasive procedure	Yes	Usually not or relatively not
Possible to diagnose thyroid carcinoma	Yes	Yes, but not follicular carcinoma
Possible to diagnose invasion	Yes	Not for certain, but presumptively
Cost	Expensive	Cheaper
Speed	Slow	Fast

■ HIV and surgery

Why should a surgeon know something about HIV infection?

- General reasons
  - Risk of transmission of infection from an infected patient to the surgeon and other staff
  - Preoperatively in outpatients or the ward
  - At operation because of complicating factors
  - Postoperatively from dressings, drains and other fluids
  - From a surgeon or staff member infected with HIV to a patient
  - Iatrogenically
    - ◆ Unscreened blood used for transfusion transmitting HIV, hepatitis B virus, hepatitis C virus, CMV
  - Management of the malnourished patient
- Specific reasons
  - The need to manage patients with HIV who have neoplasms, CNS diseases and other site specific conditions

What infections are characteristically found in patients with HIV in addition to HIV itself?

- Herpes zoster, herpes simplex infections
- Tuberculosis, *Mycobacterium avium intracellular* infection (MAI)
- Candidiasis
- *Pneumocystis carinii* infection (now called *Pneumocystis jiroveci*)

- *Toxoplasma gondii* infection
- Cryptosporidiosis
- CMV infection

Why do patients with AIDS become malnourished?
- AIDS-specific wasting
- Malabsorption and diarrhoea, nausea and vomiting
- Increased metabolic rate
- Intercurrent infections, especially pulmonary and oropharyngeal candidiasis
- Antibiotic therapy

What neoplasms are characteristic in patients with AIDS?
- Lymphomas, especially non-Hodgkin's lymphoma
- Cervical carcinoma
- Kaposi's lesion (this is now considered a reactive vascular condition related to herpes simplex virus type 8 rather than a true neoplasm)

Other than those related to infections and neoplasms, what surgical specialties are also important?
- *Ophthalmic surgeons*: ocular vasculopathy, retinal haemorrhage, CMV retinitis, Kaposi's lesion of conjunctiva
- *Neurosurgeons*: toxoplasmosis, neuropathies, AIDS specific dementia
- *Cardiothoracic surgeons*: heart muscle disease from drug therapy

Hormones and neoplasia

In what ways are hormones related to neoplasia?

- Hormones cause neoplasia
- Neoplasms secrete hormones
- Neoplasms may be hormone dependent
- Neoplasms may be treated by hormones or their antagonists

Which hormones cause neoplasms?

- Tamoxifen causes endometrial adenocarcinoma, because tamoxifen is a partial oestrogen agonist which blocks the oestrogen receptors in the breast but stimulates the endometrial oestrogen receptors
- Oestrogen causes ovarian and breast carcinoma
- Methylated steroid hormones, especially testosterone derivatives, cause liver neoplasms

Which neoplasms secrete hormones?

- Eutopic secretion from tumours of tissues that normally secrete hormones
  - Adrenal adenoma
  - Adrenal carcinoma
  - Ovarian neoplasms
    - Granulosa cell tumour
    - Thecoma
  - Thyroid neoplasms
  - Pituitary neoplasms

- Ectopic secretion from tumours of tissues that do not normally secrete hormones
  - Carcinoid of small intestine, bronchus, elsewhere
  - Atypical carcinoid
  - Neuroendocrine tumour elsewhere

Which neoplasms are dependent on hormones for growth?

- Papillary carcinoma of thyroid is dependent on thyroid-stimulating hormone (TSH)
- Breast carcinoma is dependent on oestrogen

Which neoplasms can be usefully treated with hormones, hormone partial agonists or hormone antagonists to decrease growth?

- Breast carcinoma with tamoxifen
- Endometrial carcinoma with progestogens
- Prostate carcinoma with antiandrogens, gonadotrophin-releasing agent partial agonists
- Thyroid carcinoma with thyroxine, particularly papillary and follicular types

■ Hydatid disease

What is hydatid disease?

A chronic zoonosis cause by the tapeworm *Ecchinococcus* in which man is the accidental intermediate host.

List its causes.

- *Ecchinococcus granulosus*: causes hydatid disease
- *Ecchinococcus vogeli, cadadiensis, borealis*: cause hydatid disease
- *Ecchinococcus multilocularis*: causes pulmonary hydatid disease

What are its geography and mode of transmission?

- Europe
  - Definitive host: dogs, foxes, ruminants
  - Intermediate host: rats
- America
  - Definitive host: foxes, ruminants
  - Intermediate host: rats
- Asia
  - Definitive host: dogs, cats
  - Intermediate host: rats
- Africa
  - Definitive host: dogs
  - Intermediate host: rats

How are the cysts distributed?

- Liver in 65%: cysts up to 20 cm in diameter, often multiple, especially in the right lobe

- Lungs in 20%: cysts up to 20 cm in diameter, often multiple
- Peritoneal cavity in 8%: cysts up to 50 cm in diameter
- Kidneys in 3%: cysts up to 15 cm in diameter

What are the histological features?
- Three layers of the cyst wall
  - Outer layer of host fibrous tissue
  - Middle layer of hyaline protein from parasite
  - Inner layer of germinal tissues with scolices of progeny
- Daughter cysts within the main cyst

What are the clinical features?
- Tend to present late
- Right hypochondrial pain
- Rarely jaundice
- Skin rashes, pruritus

How is hydatid disease investigated?
- Full blood count (FBC): eosinophilia is common
- Serology for specific assay
- Casoni test (historic nowadays)
- Radiology and ultrasound
- Laparotomy with care not to rupture: associated with dissemination and anaphylactic shock
- *Not* aspiration

▣ Hypercalcaemia

What is the normal serum calcium level?

2.15–2.55 mmol/l with small variations among laboratories.
Above 2.60 mmol/l is usually accepted as hypercalcaemia.

What are the commonest causes of hypercalcaemia?

- Parathyroid disease: about 1% of the population in the UK has mild primary hyperparathyroidism
- Malignancy
  - Metastases (whether osteosclerotic or osteolytic)
  - Hypercalcaemia in myeloma, leukaemia, lymphoma
  - Tumours making large amounts of parathyroid hormone-related protein (PTHrp)
    - PTHrp is a normal constituent of all cells that is secreted as a local communicator among them
    - The amount in the circulation increases when there is widespread metastatic carcinoma, causing demineralisation of bones generally
  - Tumours making parathyroid-like hormone, such as oat cell carcinoma
- Other endocrine diseases
  - Addison's disease
  - Pheochromocytoma
  - Severe hyperthyroidism
- Iatrogenic
  - Drugs: lithium, thiazides, oestrogens, androgen, tamoxifen
  - Excess vitamin A or vitamin D

- Prolonged immobilisation such as in intensive care unit (ICU) or high-dependency unit (HDU) patients and in patients with Paget's disease of bone
- Familial and congenital causes
  - Familial hypocalciuric hypercalcaemia
  - Hypophosphatasia
  - Idiopathic hypercalcaemia of infancy
- Other causes
  - Diseases with very numerous granulomas, the macrophages of which change the inactive early forms of vitamin D into very active metabolites by hydroxylation at the 25th and 1st positions
    - Sarcoidosis
    - Tuberculosis

What are the clinically important effects of hypercalcaemia?

- Bones
  - Bone pain
  - Joint pain
  - Pathological fractures
- Moans
  - Depression and confusion
  - Neuroses and psychoses
  - Fatigue, lethargy, muscle weakness
  - Pruritus
- Groans
  - Constipation
  - Peptic ulcers

- Anorexia and weight loss
- Nausea and vomiting
- Pancreatitis
- Stones
  - Polyuria and polydipsia
  - Renal calculi
  - Nephrocalcinosis
  - Renal failure
- Overtones: in longstanding cases
  - Hypertension
  - Heart block, shortened QT interval and depressed T-waves
  - Corneal calcification
  - Metastatic calcification elsewhere

■ Hyperparathyroidism

What does hyperparathyroidism mean?
Excess secretion of parathyroid hormone.

How is hyperparathyroidism classified?
Primary, secondary and tertiary.

In primary hyperparathyroidism, where is the primary defect?
In the parathyroid glands: 85% adenoma, 15% hyperplasia, $\ll$1% carcinoma.

What is the effect on the circulating calcium concentration in primary hyperparathyroidism?
The serum calcium concentration goes up, phosphate down.

In secondary hyperparathyroidism, what is the stimulus that produces this secondary effect?
Hypocalcaemia, as a result of abnormalities:
- In the kidneys
  - Decreased metabolism of vitamin D precursor to 1,25-dihydroxy vitamin D
  - Decreased renal resorption of calcium
- In the diet
  - Decreased vitamin D ingestion
- Physiologically
  - Decreased exposure to sunlight decreasing formation of cholecalciferol in skin

- Vitamin D inhibits transcription of parathyroid hormone (PTH) normally: decrease in vitamin D therefore causes secondary hyperparathyroidism
- In pregnancy
  - Increased demands

What is the circulating calcium concentration in secondary hyperparathyroidism?

The serum calcium concentration is low and phosphate is high, which stimulate the hyperparathyroidism as a secondary effect.

Tertiary hyperparathyroidism occurs under what conditions?

Autonomous adenoma supervening after years of secondary hyperparathyroidism.

What is the effect on the circulating calcium concentration in tertiary hyperparathyroidism?

Serum calcium concentration rises, phosphate falls.

Give some complications of primary hyperparathyroidism.

- Bone disease
  - Pathological fractures
  - "Brown tumour" of bone
- Psychiatric effects
- Abdominal pain
- Renal effects
  - Calculi, nephrocalcinosis
- Associated with multiple endocrine adenopathy (MEA) I and IIa (and occasionally with MEA IIb)

■ Hyperplasia and hypertrophy

How are hyperplasia and hypertrophy defined?
- *Hyperplasia*: an increase in the size of an organ or tissue because of an increase in the *number* of its cells.
- *Hypertrophy*: an increase in the size of an organ or tissue because of an increase in the *size* of its cells.

Are hyperplasia and hypertrophy mutually exclusive?
No. They both occur in:
- Graves' disease
- Adrenal hyperplasia
- Prostatic enlargement

How are hyperplasia and hypertrophy classified?
Physiological and pathological:

	Hyperplasia	Hypertrophy
Physiological	Breasts in pregnancy	Uterus in pregnancy
	Thyroid in pregnancy	Skeletal muscles with
	Pituitary in pregnancy	exercise
Pathological	Overstimulation	Overstimulation
	• Graves' disease	• Graves' disease
	• Adrenals in Cushing's disease	• Cardiomyopathies
	• Endometrium in oestrogen excess	• Congenital muscular dystrophies

▮ Hypersensitivity reactions

How is hypersensitivity classified?

Into types I to IV hypersensitivity reactions (some authors regard autoimmune interactions as a type V, such as the stimulatory antibodies in Graves' disease).

What is a type I hypersensitivity reaction?

- Linkage of two IgE molecules by an antigen results in
  - Breakdown products of arachidonic acid being formed such as leucotrienes and prostaglandins
  - Release of mast cell contents such as histamine, 5-hydroxytryptamine, heparin, eosinophil chemokines and platelet-activating factor
- Diseases caused include
  - Atopic eczema
  - Extrinsic asthma
  - Allergic rhinitis

What is a type II hypersensitivity reaction?

- Antibody in the serum reacts specifically against a tissue component resulting in cell death, either by complement action, destruction by natural killer T-cells or phagocytosis by macrophages
- Diseases caused include
  - Complement-mediated haemolysis, as in blood transfusion reactions and autoimmune haemolysis
  - Iatrogenic toxicity to red cells and platelets by drugs

What is a type III hypersensitivity reaction?

- Formation of intermediate-sized immune complexes that activate complement and platelets and cause tissue damage from ischaemia from thrombus formation, membrane attack complexes, and enzyme release from inflammatory cells
- Large immune complexes are removed by macrophages; small complexes are filtered out by the glomeruli, so only intermediate ones cause disease and circulate (serum sickness) or are found in tissues (Arthus reaction)

What is a type IV hypersensitivity reaction?

- Tissue injury characteristically associated with granuloma formation and T-lymphocyte sensitisation, a reaction to
  - Micro-organisms such as mycobacteria and fungi
  - Dermatitis from beryllium, nickel and other irritants
  - Late stage rejection of organ transplants

▉ Immunisation

How is the induction of immunity classified?
Active and passive, each divided into natural and artificial.

Give examples.
- *Natural active immunity*: following infection
- *Artificial active immunity*: following vaccination
- *Natural passive immunity*: transplacental transfer of IgG protects for first 6 months of life
- *Artificial passive immunity*: injection of preformed antibody derived from man or animals

What are the different types of vaccine and their efficacy?
- Live-attenuated organisms result in:
  - Long-lasting immunity
  - Potential danger in immunocompromised patients
- Killed organisms result in:
  - Smaller immune response, usually boosters are required
- Toxoid:
  - To prevent not infection but the effects of toxin that results from infection
  - Tetanus toxoid does not prevent infection by *Clostridium tetani*
- Other bacterial constituents:
  - Surface polysaccharides
  - Proteins

Give examples of vaccination using live-attenuated and killed organisms.

- Live-attenuated
  - BCG for tuberculosis
  - Sabine vaccine for polio
  - MMR for measles, mumps and rubella
- Killed
  - Typhoid (now being replaced by live attenuated vaccine)
  - Cholera
  - Pertussis vaccine for *Bordatella pertussis* infection (whooping cough)

When is passive immunity used?

For patients exposed to HBsAg-positive blood, immuno-compromised patients with shingles, and rarely for botulism and rabies.

■ Immunoglobulins

What is the generic structure of an immunoglobulin?
- Antigen-binding sites as part of the light- and heavy-chain variable regions
- Complement activation sites as part of the heavy chains
- Immune adherence, a property of the constant regions
- The heavy chains determine the class of immunoglobulin: γ in IgG, α in IgA, μ in IgM, δ in IgD, ε in IgE
- Light chains are κ or λ irrespective of the immunoglobulin class

What is the structure and function of IgG?
- The most important quantitatively
- Monomeric
- Multiple IgG molecules must bind to a bacterium for phagocytosis by polymorphs
- Bind also to killer T-cells
- Neutralises toxins
- Activates complement (needs two molecules of IgG close together)
- Crosses the placenta (the only immunoglobulin to do so)

What is the structure and function of IgA?
- Present in secretions of the gastrointestinal tract (GIT), respiratory tract, lachrymal and salivary glands, breasts and bile
- Heavier than IgG

- Dimer with a J-chain linkage and a secretory unit that is needed to transport it across epithelial cells
- Inhibits adherence of micro-organisms to mucosal surfaces
- Activates complement

What is the structure and function of IgM?
- The largest immunoglobulin
- Pentamer held together by a J-chain as in IgA
- Multiple-binding sites and a tendency to form large complexes that precipitate
- Most effective immunoglobulin at activating complement

What is the structure and function of IgE?
- Monomer bound to mast cell membranes
- When two molecules are cross linked by antigen, histamine, leucotrienes and eosinophil chemotactic factors are released
- Activates complement

▪ Immunohistochemistry

How does an immunostaining technique differ from a haematoxylin and eosin (H&E) stain?

Immunostaining gives an indication of what a cell constituent is:

- Presence of cytokeratin, which may indicate that a tumour is a carcinoma
- Presence of hormones in the tumour cells:
  - *Adrenocorticotropic hormone (ACTH)*: in corticotrophs
  - *Human growth hormone (hGH)*: in somatotrophs
  - *Prolactin (PRL)*: in lactotrophs
  - *Thyroid-stimulating hormone (TSH)*: in thyrotrophs
  - *Follicle-stimulating hormone (FSH)*: in gonadotrophs
  - *Luteinising hormone (LH)*: in gonadotrophs
  - *Inhibin*: in granulosa cell tumour of the ovary
  - *Beta human chorionic gonadotropin (βhCG)*: in trophoblastic tumours

What are the difficulties in interpreting immunostains?

- Cytokeratins are positive in epithelial neoplasms but can occasionally be positive in connective tissue neoplasms such as leiomyoma.
- Edge effects, in which there is staining at the periphery of the tissue samples, can lead to false-positive staining and misinterpretation.

- Negative immunostaining might mean not that the tissue does not make the antigen stained for but that the tissue has made the antigen (such as a hormone) and has actively secreted all of it and so retains none that can be demonstrated on immunostaining.

Immunohistochemistry

■ Infections in compromised patients

How may a patient become compromised so that he or she develops an infection?

- Patients who are immunocompromised
  - Congenital
    - Bruton-type hypogammaglobulinaemia
    - Cell-mediated (Di George-type)
    - Combined (Swiss-type with agammaglobulinaemia and stem cell deficiency)
    - Deficiency of neutrophil function in chronic granulomatous disease
  - Acquired
    - AIDS
    - Steroid therapy, other immunosuppressive drugs such as cytotoxics and transplant-related therapy
    - Diabetes (also because of glucose as culture medium in urine and on skin)
- Patients in unusual circumstances
  - Catheterisation
    - Urethral/vesical
    - Intravenous, such as short catheters and Hickman lines
  - Intensive care units
    - Catheterisation
    - Administration of oxygen especially with humidification
    - Active ventilation

- Patients with prostheses
  - Orthopaedic
    - Hip and knee joints especially
  - Artificial heart valves

What are the sources of infection in these patients?

- Endogenous from normal flora
  - Colonic bacteria causing septicaemia
  - *Candida* in the oesophagus and GI system causing invasive candidiasis
- Exogenous infection
  - Infections that are not normally injurious in normal people
    - Nocardiasis
    - *Pneumocystis carinii* infection (now called *Pneumocystis jiroveci*)
    - Cytomegalovirus
  - Infections normally injurious but more likely to be acquired by compromised patients
    - Tuberculosis
    - Toxoplasmosis
  - Infections in transplanted tissues
    - Cytomegalovirus

■ Inflammatory mediators

How are inflammatory mediators classified?
- Substances stored in cells irrespective of need and released when required:
  - Histamine
  - Serotonin
- Substances synthesised in cells as required when inflammatory events dictate
  - Substances derived from arachidonic acid:
    - Leucotrienes
    - Prostaglandins
    - Cytokines
- Cascades that pre-exist and are activated as part of the inflammatory response
  - Clotting cascade and its fibrinolytic component
  - Complement cascade, a series of plasma proteins that act as
    - Opsonins
    - Chemoattractants
    - Anaphylactic agents
    - Effectors of membrane lysis
  - Kinin cascade

What are the prime plasma-derived mediators in acute inflammation?
- Fibrin-related peptides, plasmin
- Kallikrein, bradykinin
- C3a, C5a

■ Intracranial haemorrhage

What does the term *intracranial haemorrhage* encompass?

- bleeding in any of the potential spaces, spaces or solid structures housed in the cranial cavity

How is intracranial haemorrhage classified?

By site, into:

- Extradural
- Subdural
- Subarachnoid
- Intracerebral
- Intraventricular

What are the pathological features and anatomical disturbances of intracranial haemorrhage?

- Extradural haemorrhage
  - Usually from tearing of the middle meningeal artery as a consequence of fracture of the squamous temporal bone
  - Occasionally from tearing an intracranial venous sinus
  - Haematoma limited by arterial spasm and attachments of the dura at the suture lines
  - A space-occupying lesion which might result in downward pressure with herniation
- Subdural haemorrhage
  - Rupture of communicating veins (bridging veins) between the brain and the dural venous sinuses

- Not limited by muscular spasm (veins have little muscle in their walls) and not limited by dural attachments, so more diffuse over the surface of the brain and less of a space-occupying lesion
- Subarachnoid haemorrhage
    - Classically from rupture of a berry aneurysm in the circle of Willis
    - Not causatively associated with hypertension
    - Associated with polycystic disease of the liver, pancreas, kidneys, spleen
- Intracerebral haemorrhage
    - Classically from
        - rupture of a microaneurysm (Charcot-Bouchard aneurysm) on the lenticulostriate artery
        - thrombosis and rupture of a cerebral artery
        - embolus to a cerebral artery
    - Involves the internal capsule in most cases and results in stroke
    - Also caused by tracking from a subarachnoid haemorrhage into the underlying cerebral tissues, in which case a stroke would be less likely
- Intraventricular haemorrhage
    - Any cause of an intracerebral haemorrhage with tracking of blood into the ventricles
    - Haemorrhage from intraventricular structures and tumours of them

■ Ischaemia and infarction

What are ischaemia and infarction?

Ischaemia is an abnormal reduction of the blood supply to or drainage from an organ or tissue. Infarction is the result of cessation of the blood supply to or drainage from an organ or tissue.

How do you classify the causes of ischaemia and infarction?

- Local causes
  - Arterial obstruction
    - Thrombus
    - Embolus
    - Atheroma in vessels down to 1 mm diameter
    - Pressure from outside the vessel (e.g. ligation, tourniquet)
    - Spasm
  - Venous obstruction
    - Thrombus
    - Pressure from
      - ▲ Torsion or volvulus
      - ▲ Strangulation of hernia
      - ▲ Intussusception
    - Stasis from varicose veins
  - Capillary obstruction
    - Vasculitis from
      - ▲ Meningococcal septicaemia
      - ▲ Drug eruptions

- ◆ Obstruction in
  - ▲ Sickle cell disease
  - ▲ Malaria
  - ▲ Cryoglobulinaemia
  - ▲ Fat embolism
  - ▲ Caisson disease with nitrogen bubbles
  - ▲ Frostbite
- ◆ External pressure in decubitus such as bedsores
- General causes
  - ■ Causes of hypoxaemia
    - ◆ Decreased cardiac output
      - ▲ Myocardial ischaemia
      - ▲ Myocardial infarction
      - ▲ Heart block
  - ■ Anaemia
  - ■ Ventilation/perfusion (V/Q) defect

What factors determine the extent of ischaemic damage in arterial obstruction?

- Tissue involved – the brain and heart are much more susceptible than skeletal muscle and skin
- Speed of onset
- Degree of obstruction of the arterial lumen
- Presence of collaterals and of disease in them
- Level of oxygenation of the blood supplying the ischaemic tissue
- Presence of concomitant heart failure
- State of the microcirculation, as in diabetes mellitus

■ Ischaemia–reperfusion injury

What is ischaemia–reperfusion injury?

- The damage that results from re-introduction of oxygen to an area of ischaemia:
  - Generation of oxygen free radicals ("reactive-oxygen species")
  - Cellular damage from:
    - Lipid peroxidation
    - DNA strand breaks
    - Protein inactivation
  - Prostaglandin activation
  - Complement activation
  - Leucocyte–endothelial cell adhesion
  - Platelet–leucocyte aggregation
  - Increased microvascular permeability
- May affect any reperfused tissues:
  - Liver during liver surgery and transplantation
  - Heart after cardiopulmonary bypass
  - Muscles in compartment syndrome and after prolonged tourniquet use

What are the effects of the cell damage?

- Local effects
  - Leakage of fluid through damaged endothelium causing oedema
  - Muscle cell breakdown
  - Further damage from capillary occlusion resulting from the increasing pressure

- Systemic effects
  - Hyperkalaemia
  - Leucocytosis
  - Increase in circulating creatine kinase

How is ischaemia–reperfusion injury treated?

With difficulty. Inhibition of the inflammation resulting from the reperfusion might inhibit important protective physiological responses or result in immunosuppression. Strategies include:

- Ischaemic preconditioning where appropriate
- Anti-oxidant therapy
- Controlled reperfusion
- Indomethacin to inhibit prostaglandin activity

■ Jaundice I: bilirubin handling

How is bilirubin formed and handled in the body?

- Bilirubin is derived from:
  - Haem from red cells
  - A little from cytochrome enzymes
  - A little probably from myoglobin
- Red cells are degraded in the spleen principally
  - Unconjugated bilirubin is insoluble in water and so is carried in plasma strongly bound to albumin
- In the liver, bilirubin is conjugated with glucuronide
  - Bilirubin glucuronide is excreted in bile bound to cholesterol, lipids and bile salts as micelles
- In the small bowel, bilirubin diglucuronide is not metabolised
- In the colon, it is metabolised by being unconjugated by bacterial glucuronidases and then reduced to stercobilinogen
- Stercobilinogen is excreted in the faeces as stercobilin
- The small amount of stercobilinogen pigment that is absorbed by the colon is handled by recycling by the liver and excretion in bile
- The tiny amount of stercobilinogen that escapes into the systemic plasma is excreted as urobilinogen which is colourless

Give some clinically important differences between conjugated and unconjugated bilirubin.

- Conjugated bilirubin can be excreted in urine; unconjugated bilirubin cannot escape through the glomerulus because of strong binding to albumin. The excess of unconjugated bilirubin in haemolytic states is therefore not able to escape and so the patient develops "acholuric" jaundice without bilirubin in the urine.

- Excess unconjugated bilirubin can swamp the capacity of albumin to carry it and then, especially in neonates, becomes attached to lipid-rich areas in the brain such as the basal ganglia causing kernicterus.
- Obstructive jaundice, in which the bilirubin is conjugated, is never associated with kernicterus.

Jaundice II: classification and tests

How is jaundice classified?

Into haemolytic and other pre-hepatic causes, hepatocellular causes and obstructive causes

- In haemolytic jaundice, in terms of bilirubin and its metabolites in the serum and urine:
  - Excess breakdown of red cells resulting in excess circulating unconjugated bilirubin
    - Excess stercobilinogen because the unconjugated bilirubin is metabolised by the liver in due course
    - Excess urobilinogen because there is more reabsorbed stercobilinogen which spills into the plasma and then urine
  - Absence in the urine of bilirubin
- In hepatocellular jaundice, in terms of bilirubin and its metabolites:
  - Excess of both conjugated and unconjugated bilirubin because of hepatocyte failure to conjugate
  - Failure to excrete the bilirubin that has been conjugated
  - Enzyme deficiencies, especially in children and young adults, called Gilbert's syndrome, Dubin–Johnson syndrome, Crigler–Najjar syndrome
- In obstructive jaundice, in terms of bilirubin and its metabolites:
  - Excess of conjugated bilirubin in the plasma because bilirubin cannot be excreted in bile

- Excess of conjugated bilirubin in the urine because bilirubin cannot be excreted in bile
- Decreased amounts of stercobilinogen pigment in faeces because bilirubin cannot be excreted in bile
- Pale faeces because bile pigments (stercobilinogen and stercobilin) are low or absent

What simple serological tests are relevant in the investigation of a patient with jaundice?

- Full blood count (FBC), film, reticulocyte count, erythrocyte sedimentation rate (ESR), C-reactive protein
- Clotting investigations
- Routine liver function tests including albumin and total protein measurements
- Virological investigations
- Autoantibody screen

■ Lung cancer

Is lung carcinoma a surgically important disease?

The trigger for surgical intervention is whether the tumour is a small cell (oat cell) carcinoma or not. Of all bronchial and lung carcinomas, two-thirds are inoperable irrespective of tumour type.

If the tumour is a small cell carcinoma, operative surgery is inappropriate even when the tumour is small – the presumption is that the tumour has metastasised by the time of diagnosis and so cannot be cured or alleviated by surgical excision of the primary carcinoma.

Small cell (oat cell) carcinoma:
- About 20% of all bronchial/lung cancers
- Commoner in men
- Usually a small tumour on presentation
- Metastasises early and widely
- Hilar location
- May be associated with paraneoplastic syndromes
- First described at St. Thomas's Hospital, London in 1932. Before that it was thought to be lymphoma of lung

Which types of lung carcinoma can be treated by operative surgery?

The types of lung carcinoma (bronchial or parenchymal) that can be treated by surgical excision include:
- Squamous cell carcinoma
  - About 35% of all bronchial/lung cancers
  - Commoner in men

- Usually a large tumour on presentation
- Hilar location related to large bronchi
- May be associated with bronchiectasis
- Adenocarcinoma
  - About 40% of all bronchial/lung cancers
  - Peripheral location
  - Commoner in women
  - May be associated with scarring
  - Must distinguish adenocarcinoma arising in the lung from metastatic adenocarcinoma

What is the aetiology of lung cancer?

- Smoking tobacco
  - Tar in cigarette smoke contains
    - Polycyclic hydrocarbons
    - Nitrosamines, nicotine, cadmium, nickel
  - The gas phase of cigarette smoke contains
    - Free radicals
    - Nitric oxide, nickel compounds, vinyl chloride
- Asbestos
- Arsenic, used by vineyard workers
- Ionising radiation
- Vaporised metals in smelting works

Lymphadenopathy: classification

- Non-neoplastic
  - By histological features:
    - Non-specific, acute and chronic (acute lymphadenitis is rarely biopsied)
      - Follicular enlargement
      - Sinus histiocytosis
      - Dilatation of subcapsular sinus
    - Specific
      - Granulomatous
        - Tuberculosis, sarcoidosis, fungal infections
        - Draining a malignant neoplasm (without metastasis)
      - Dermatopathic
      - AIDS changes
      - Toxoplasmal changes
      - Cat-scratch fever
  - By causation:
    - Infective
      - Organism: viruses and bacteria principally
      - Specific infections such as infectious mononucleosis
    - Inflammatory, non-infective
      - Rheumatoid arthritis, systemic lupus erythematosus
      - Ulcerative colitis and Crohn's disease

- - ▲ Draining a malignant neoplasm (without metastasis)
  - ■ By anatomical group:
    - ◆ Posterior triangle of neck, submental, inguinal, internal iliac, etc.
- Neoplastic
  - ■ Metastatic spread to lymph nodes
    - ◆ Breast, bronchus, kidney, thyroid, prostate
    - ◆ Other carcinomas
    - ◆ Rarely sarcomas
  - ■ Primary neoplasms of lymph nodes
    - ◆ Lymphoma
      - ▲ Hodgkin's lymphoma
      - ▲ Non-Hodgkin's lymphoma (NHL)
    - ◆ Primary nodal Kaposi's sarcoma (probably not a true neoplasm)
    - ◆ Lymphangiosarcoma

■ Lymphoedema

Impairment of lymphatic drainage leading to accumulation of extracellular fluid in the tissues.

Classify lymphoedema.

- *Primary lymphoedema*, a developmental abnormality. Milroy's disease is an autosomal-dominant condition:
  - Some patients have too few lymphatics from aplasia or hypoplasia
  - Some patients have normal numbers of varicose lymphatics that do not contract properly
- *Secondary lymphoedema* as a result of:
  - Infection
    - Repeated acute bacterial infections in people who walk barefoot
    - Chronic
      - Filariasis: *Wuchereria bancrofti* infection, elephantiasis
      - Tuberculosis
      - Fungal infections: cryptosporidiosis, sporotrichosis
  - Injury
    - Iatrogenic
      - Lymphadenectomy
      - Radiotherapy
    - Burns
  - Neoplasia
    - Blockage of lymphatics and nodal drainage by metastatic neoplasms

What are the clinical aspects?

- Tightness, heaviness and fatigue in affected limb
- Thickening of skin, especially the keratin layer
- Gross distortion of anatomy in severe cases, elephantiasis
- Paraesthesiae
- Tenderness in popliteal fossa, groin, axilla
- Heat intolerance
- Tendency to develop infections such as cellulitis

Lymphoma I: Hodgkin's disease

Why is Hodgkin's disease differentiated from the other lymphoma types?

- The clinical and pathological features are unlike those of non-Hodgkin's lymphoma and are characteristic enough to make Hodgkin's disease a recognisable entity
- The characteristic cell is the Reed-Sternberg cell. Any lymphoma that has Reed-Sternberg cells is Hodgkin's disease. A Reed-Sternberg cell is a B lymphocyte modified at an immature stage

What is the cause of Hodgkin's disease?

- Unknown but Ebstein–Barr virus (EBV) is a strong contender
  - A history of glandular fever is associated with an increased risk of Hodgkin's disease
  - Patients with Hodgkin's disease have a higher prevalence of antibodies against EBV than would be expected by chance
  - Reed-Sternberg cells have a genomic sequence of EBV in their nuclei. A protein gene product of EBV is also found in Reed-Sternberg cells

How is Hodgkin's disease classified into histological types?

By the modified Rye classification, in order of 5-year survival:

- Lymphocyte predominance
  - About 10% of all cases of Hodgkin's disease
  - Diffuse sheets of well differentiated lymphocytes
  - Reed-Sternberg cells are present but have to be searched for

- Nodular sclerosis
  - Accounts for most cases of Hodgkin's disease, about 70%
  - Fibrous septa dividing the lymphoma cells in to nodules
  - Reed-Sternberg cells are commoner and may form *lacunar cells* by collapse of the cytoplasm on fixation
- Mixed cellularity
  - About 20% of all cases of Hodgkin's disease
  - Sheets of lymphoma cells, plasma cells, eosinophils, neutrophils and other inflammatory cell types, hence the name
  - Reed-Sternberg cells in obvious numbers
- Lymphocyte depletion
  - A very small proportion of cases of Hodgkin's disease
  - Few lymphocytes, large numbers of pleomorphic tumour cells and Reed-Sternberg cells

How is Hodgkin's disease usually staged?

By the Ann Arbor system:

- Stage 1 – one lymph node group
- Stage 2 – two or more lymph node groups on the same side of the diaphragm
- Stage 3 – lymph node groups on both sides of the diaphragm; splenic involvement is taken to be the same as nodal involvement
- Stage 4 – diffuse extranodal tissues with or without lymph node involvement

With all of the stages, there is a subclassification into A, in which the patients are symptomless, and B in which they have pyrexia, sweats and weight loss or a combination of these.

Lymphoma II: non-Hodgkin's lymphoma

Why should a surgeon know about NHL?

- A surgical patient may incidentally have NHL or be receiving treatment for one
- NHL causes immunosuppression
- Lymph node excision, splenectomy and liver wedge biopsy might be necessary (rare nowadays)
- Skin biopsy might be necessary for the diagnosis of mycosis fungoides
- A patient with Hodgkin's disease can develop NHL and so the clinical features might be confusing

How is NHL classified?

There are many classifications, and new ones being proposed as the techniques available for the investigation of the cell types involved in NHL develop. In essence, the classification of NHL involves determination of:

- Cell lineage: B-cells, T-cells, platelets
- Degree of differentiation or maturity of the cells involved
- Presence of different surface markers
- State of activation of the cells involved: activation may indicate aggressive behaviour

Chromosome abnormalities are common in NHL and it is likely in the near future that the presence of gene translocations and other genetic abnormalities in the cells of the NHL will form a part of the classification.

How is NHL classified usefully in surgical terms?

Into

- Low-grade or high-grade (indolent or aggressive)
- B- or T-lymphocyte lymphomas
  - Indolent lymphomas
    - Follicular lymphoma
    - Small lymphocytic lymphoma
    - Lymphoplasmacytic lymphoma (Waldenstrom's macroglobulinaemia)
    - Mucosa-associated lymphoid tissue (MALT) lymphoma
  - Aggressive lymphomas
    - Diffuse large cell lymphoma
    - Anaplastic large cell lymphoma
- NHL of other cell lineages
  - Plasma cell neoplasms
    - Plasmacytoma
    - Multiple myeloma
  - Histiocytoses
    - Langerhans cell histiocytosis
      - Eosinophilic granuloma
      - Hand–Schüller–Christian syndrome
      - Letterer–Siwe disease
- Named types
  - *Burkitt's lymphoma*: a B-cell lymphoma
  - *Mycosis fungoides* and *Sézary's syndrome*: T-cell lymphomas

■ Macrocytic and megaloblastic anaemia

Is a macrocyte a normal red cell precursor? Is a megaloblast a normal red cell precursor?

No and no.

What are the normal red cell precursors?

Myeloblasts, myelocytes, early normoblasts, late normoblasts, reticulocytes. Reticulocytes are anucleate large red cells that have a "reticule" (a network or meshwork) of basophilic filaments that are the remnants of RNA in the cell.

Must a patient with a macrocytic anaemia have megaloblasts?

No. Macrocytic anaemia alone can be caused by:

- Liver damage, especially as a consequence of alcohol consumption
- Thyroid disease
- Renal failure

What is a megaloblast?

- An abnormal nucleated red cell not usually found in the body
- Present in bone marrow and occasionally found in the peripheral blood
- Tetraploid or aneuploid because of deranged DNA metabolism

- Caused by deficiency of vitamin B_{12} (cobalamin) or folate or both
- Nuclear abnormality is present in all cells that have nuclei, and so can find nuclear changes on cervical cytology, sputum cytology
- In vitamin B_{12} and folate deficiency the red cells miss a division in their maturation and so are large.

What are folate and vitamin B_{12} used for in the body?

Tetrahydrofolate, the reduced form, is used in all cells in the formation of methionine from homocysteine. The reaction between homocysteine and methylated tetrahydrofolate requires vitamin B_{12} as a co-enzyme to produce methionine and tetrahydrofolate. Methionine is essential for the formation of many proteins and nucleotides.

How much vitamin B_{12} and folate are found in body stores?

- About 3 months stores of folate in the liver
- Over 3 years stores of vitamin B_{12} in the liver, which is why pregnant women are given folate supplements but not vitamin B_{12} supplements

What are the causes of vitamin B_{12} deficiency?

- Absence of intrinsic factor
  - Pernicious anaemia because antibodies against parietal cells reduce secretion
  - Partial or total gastrectomy
- Absence of absorption
  - Disease in the terminal ileum such as Crohn's disease

What are the causes of folate deficiency?

- Pregnancy
  - Increased demands from the fetus
- Dietary deficiency
  - Nutritional
  - Behavioural as in vegans
- Drugs which have an antifolate action, such as methotrexate

■ Macrophages

What are the functions of a macrophage?

- Migration as the response to lymphokines
- Phagocytosis, via a process of
  - *Opsonisation*: making particles such as bacteria more easily captured and ingested by phagocytes
  - Surface receptors for C3b and IgG which opsonise particles of different sizes, some large. When the particle is larger than a single macrophage, fusion of macrophages may occur
- Antigen presentation to CD4 cells
- Digestion
  - Secondary lysosome enzymes and respiratory burst
  - Not all organisms are digestible; mycobacteria, listeria, toxoplasma, chlamydia and rickettsia can survive
- Multinucleate giant cell formation, which may be of several types
  - Foreign body type with haphazard nuclei
  - Langhans' type with a cap or horseshoe of nuclei – the result of longevity rather than specifically of mycobacterial infection
  - Touton type in xanthoma and xanthelasma
- Metabolism: vitamin D precursors are hydroxylated to the active form, accounting for the finding of hypercalcaemia in sarcoidosis

- Secretion
  - Of interleukins, transforming growth factors, tumour necrosis factors, prostaglandins, leucotrienes and hence tissue damage, scarring, lymphocyte activation
  - Characteristically after taking on an epithelioid appearance, in which the cells accumulate cytoplasm with large amounts of rough endoplasmic reticulum (RER) and a large Golgi and so appear plump and eosinophilic

Define a granuloma.

- Histologically, an apparently expansile localised collection of macrophages
- Immunologically, a collection of activated macrophages surrounded by a collar of lymphocytes

Give some causes of granulomas.

- Infective agents
  - Mycobacterial diseases, especially TB and tuberculoid leprosy
  - Fungi, actinomycosis, syphilis
- Beryllium, silica and other inorganic indigestible and foreign materials
- Sarcoidosis
- Crohn's disease
- Malignancy, in the primary or in lymph nodes draining the site with or without metastatic involvement

■ Malignant tumours: local spread

What factors determine the extent of local spread of a malignant tumour, at least for a time?

- Tumour factors
  - The tumour type (squamous cell carcinoma (SCC), adenocarcinoma, transitional cell carcinoma, undifferentiated carcinoma)
  - The tumour differentiation or grade: well, moderately or poorly differentiated or undifferentiated (anaplastic means undifferentiated – there is no distinction)
  - The site of origin, in relation to the intrinsic behaviour of the tumour irrespective of type or differentiation. For example, well-differentiated SCC of the skin will behave in a more indolent fashion than well-differentiated SCC of the bronchus or bladder
  - The presence of a fibrous capsule around the tumour (rare)
- Local factors around the tumour
  - Blood supply
  - Tissue planes
  - Tissues resistant to infiltration such as cartilage, because of lack of blood supply and secretion of inhibitors of hyaluronidase
  - Local cellular immune response to the tumour by lymphocytes, histiocytes and eosinophils

- Systemic factors
  - Humoral immune response to the tumour by circulating (and local) immunoglobulins
  - Nutrition
  - Infection

■ Malnutrition

How is malnutrition defined?
Failure to achieve normal nutritional requirements. This failure may be due to undernutrition or overnutrition. The latter is the commonest type of malnutrition in the Western world.

Classify malnutrition.
- Undernutrition
  - Too little food generally: *marasmus*
  - Too little specific ingestion of
    - Protein: *kwashiorkor*
    - Vitamins
      - Fat-soluble vitamins are stored in the body (mostly in the liver) and deficiency takes years
      - Water-soluble vitamins are not stored in large quantities and deficiencies of vitamin B, vitamin C and folic acid present relatively earlier
    - Iron
    - Iodine
    - Trace minerals
  - Available food but chronic disease resulting in malnutrition
    - Small bowel malabsorption
    - Renal failure
    - Diarrhoea
    - Infections

- Drug addiction
- Anorexia
- Overnutrition
  - Too much food generally
    - Obesity (BMI (body mass index) > 30) and morbid obesity (BMI > 40)
  - Too much specific ingestion of
    - Vitamins, especially vitamin A, niacin (vitamin B_3), pyridoxine (vitamin B_6) and vitamin D
    - Fats
  - Insufficient exercise
  - Specific diets, exclusive diets, parenteral nutrition

Which people are particularly at risk of malnutrition?

- Neonates
  - Vitamin K deficiency
  - Vitamin B_{12} deficiency in breastfed babies of vegans
- Children
  - Iron, folate, vitamin A, vitamin C, copper, zinc
- Pregnant and lactating women
  - Folate
  - Excessive alcohol intake causing
    - Fetal alcohol syndrome
    - Deficiency of magnesium, zinc, thiamine (vitamin B_1)
- People in areas of famine, extreme poverty
- The elderly
  - Iron deficiency

- Osteoporosis from relative calcium deficiency
- Osteomalacia from lack of sunlight exposure and dietary deficiency of vitamin D
- Patients with chronic disease
  - Patients who have had gastrectomy, excision of the terminal ileum and related operations
  - Patients with chronic renal failure, especially when on chronic dialysis
  - Patients with
    - chronic liver disease
    - AIDS
    - Malignant neoplasms
- People on specific diets
  - Vegetarians may develop iron deficiency
  - Vegans may develop vitamin B_{12} deficiency and calcium, iron and zinc intake tend to be low
  - Very low calorie diets
- Patients with alcohol and drug dependency
- Patients with AIDS
- People in societies in which excessive consumption of food is usual

How is malnutrition diagnosed?
- History
- Physical examination
  - Muscle bulk, strength
  - Anthropometry: caliper measurements, BMI
  - Specific changes of vitamin deficiencies

- Laboratory tests
    - Proteins: albumin, transferrin
    - Electrolytes and trace elements
    - Vitamin measurements
    - Liver function tests, renal function tests, small bowel absorption tests
    - Drug screening tests
    - Viral screening and other viral tests
    - Tumour markers

Give some examples of the surgical importance of malnutrition.

- Poor wound healing
    - Infection
    - Dehiscence of abdominal wounds in the morbidly obese
- Anaemia
- Impaired immunity, tendency to pulmonary and other infections
- Tendency to deep-vein thrombosis (DVT)
- Impaired respiratory function, anaesthetic problems

■ Melanocytes and their proliferations

What are the sites and function of melanocytes?

- Melanocytes are found in the basal layer of the epidermis, in the mucosa of the vulva, vagina and cervix, in the meninges, in the nasal mucosa, and occasionally in the palate.
- Melanocytes have clear cytoplasm and regular nuclei; little melanin is retained as it is injected via fine processes into adjacent epidermal basal cells and other adjacent cells at other sites.
- Melanocytes occur normally in a ratio of 1 to every 6–10 basal epithelial squamous cells.
  - It might appear paradoxical that melanin is delivered to basal cells away from the skin surface where damaging UV light hits.
  - This on face value would leave parabasal, intermediate and superficial cells unprotected, but the epidermal cells retain their melanin granules throughout their maturation through the thickness of the epidermis and so are protected at all stages.
- Melanin is made from the amino acid tyrosine. There are several enzymes involved, one or more of which may be congenitally absent in albinism.
- Patients with albinism have a normal distribution of melanocytes, but they are unable to synthesise melanin.

What are the non-neoplastic abnormalities of melanocytes?

- Ephelids or ephelides
  - Freckles
  - Not usually considered an abnormality, though may be very extensive in some people
  - The normal ratio of melanocytes to basal squamous cells, but a local increase in melanin production and delivery
  - Stimulated by sunlight to become more pigmented
- Lentigines
  - A lentigo is an "age-spot" or "liver-spot" particularly on the dorsum of the hands, the face and other sun-exposed areas
  - Not related to liver disease or primarily to age, though they are commoner in older people
  - Patients with Peutz–Jeghers syndrome develop lentigo simplex spots around the mouth and anus
  - An increase in the number of melanocytes relative to basal squamous cells, with the melanocytes in a flat sheet pushing the basal cells out of the way
  - Three types:
    - Lentigo simplex: normal epidermal architecture
    - Lentigo senilis: epidermal hyperplasia causing a raised lesion
    - Lentigo maligna or "Hutchinson's freckle" with melanocytic atypia which very rarely goes on to melanoma

- Naevi
  - Rounded collections of uniform melanocytes (rather than flat sheets as in lentigines)
  - May be congenital or acquired
  - When numerous might need follow-up with photographic "mole mapping" to detect small changes that might suggest development of melanoma
  - Four main types:
    - *Junctional naevus*: collections of melanocytes at the epidermodermal junction
    - *Compound naevus*: a combination of a junctional naevus and an intradermal naevus
    - *Intradermal naevus*: collections of melanocytes entirely in the dermis
    - *Blue naevus*: collections of darkly pigmented melanocytes usually in the deep dermis
  - Subtypes such as
    - *Halo naevus* with a surrounding depigmented area
    - *Swimming trunk naevus* over an extensive area of the lower back or groin which may develop melanoma

■ Melanoma

Define melanoma.

A malignant neoplasm of melanocytes. It is often called "malignant melanoma" but all melanomas are malignant; the term is never used for benign or reactive melanocytic lesions because of the danger of confusion.

Occurs on skin, in nasal passages, in the vulva and vagina, the anus and the oral cavity, the meninges and rarely elsewhere.

What are the four classical types of melanoma?

- Superficial spreading melanoma
  - Commonest
  - Increasing in incidence
  - Radial growth phase, no significant vertical growth phase
  - Commoner in Whites
- Nodular melanoma
  - Second commonest
  - Vertical growth phase, no radial growth phase
  - Commoner in Whites
  - In Blacks occurs at the junction of the sole with the pigmented skin of the foot
- Lentigo maligna melanoma
  - About 5% of melanomas
  - Develops in lentigo maligna, an in situ dysplastic melanocytic lesion
  - Radial growth phase

- Commoner in women
- Commoner in Whites
- Sun-exposed skin, especially of the face
- Slow growing, best prognosis
- Acral lentiginous melanoma (also called *acral melanoma*)
  - Rarest type, about 3% of melanomas
  - On extremities, especially the feet
  - May be subungual
  - Radial growth phase
  - Commonest type to arise in Blacks
  - Prognosis is a good provided diagnosis and treatment are early

List the risk factors for developing melanoma.

- Pre-existing melanocytic lesions
  - Dysplastic naevi: may be familial or sporadic
  - Large congenital moles: "swimming trunk" naevus, giant hairy naevus
  - Presence of lentigo maligna, Hutchinson's freckle, which might develop into lentigo maligna melanoma
  - Large numbers of apparently typical naevi
- Excessive exposure to sunlight, especially with burning, related to skin type
  - Type 1: dark brown or black hair, chalk-white skin, never tans, always burns
  - Type 2: red or fair hair, ruddy skin, tans with difficulty, often burns
  - Type 3: dark or fair hair, light brown skin, tans easily, sometimes burns

- Type 4: Mediterranean olive skin, tans easily, almost never burns
- Type 5: dark skin characteristic of the Indian subcontinent and parts of South America, tans easily.
- Type 6: very dark skin characteristic of equatorial Africa, tans easily
- Immunodeficiency
- Previous melanoma irrespective of any of the above
- Age: melanoma is very rare in children

What are the two main staging schemes for melanoma?

- Clark's levels
  - Level 1: tumour cells only within the epidermis
  - Level 2: tumour cells invade the papillary dermis
  - Level 3: tumour cells reach the junction between the papillary and the reticular dermis
  - Level 4: tumour cells invade the reticular dermis
  - Level 5: tumour cells invade the subcutis
- Breslow thickness
  - Measured in millimetres from the granular layer of the overlying epidermis to the deepest identifiable tumour cell
  - Metastasis is uncommon if the Breslow thickness is below 1 mm

List some prognostic features.

- Presence of a vertical growth phase (i.e. of nodular melanoma)
- Clark's level

- Breslow thickness
- Presence of nodal metastases
- Presence of ulceration
- Site of the tumour: for a given Breslow thickness, tumours on extremities have a worse prognosis
- Sex: men generally have a worse prognosis
- Age: older patients generally have a worse prognosis
- Histological features of the tumour irrespective of the above
  - Large tumour volume
  - High mitotic count
  - Satellite nodules

What chromosomal changes occur reliably in melanoma?

- The three types of melanoma with a radial growth phase have predictable abnormalities on chromosome 6
- Nodular melanoma has predictable abnormalities on chromosomes 1, 6 and 7
- Chromosome 9 is abnormal in about half of melanomas, especially those with a familial distribution
  - This is a deletion of p16, a growth-inhibitor gene which acts directly on one of the cyclin-dependent kinases which drives the cell cycle
  - Deletion of p16 is a common finding in other malignant neoplasms such as colonic carcinoma and neuroblastoma

■ Metaplasia

What is the definition of metaplasia?
A change of one fully differentiated cell type into another fully differentiated cell type.

How is metaplasia classified?
Into epithelial and connective tissue metaplasia.

Give some examples of epithelial metaplasia.
- Squamous metaplasia
  - By far the commonest
    - Endocervix
    - Bronchi
    - Bladder, renal pelvicalyceal system
    - Prostate, especially after treatment with antiandrogens
- Glandular or columnar cell metaplasia
  - Intestinal metaplasia in the stomach, usually associated with infection with *Helicobacter pylori*
  - Barrett's oesophagus which is lined by metaplastic intestinal or sometimes gastric mucosa
  - Pyloric metaplasia in the gall bladder related to gall stones
  - Apocrine metaplasia characteristically found in the breast (the breast developmentally is a modified *eccrine* sweat gland, and so the finding of apocrine change is true metaplasia)

Give three examples of connective tissue metaplasia.

- Osseous metaplasia in
  - Bladder
  - Bronchi, tracheopathia osteoplastica
  - Scars
- Chondroid metaplasia in
  - Scars
- Myeloid metaplasia in
  - Liver
  - Spleen
  - Lymph nodes

What is the significance of metaplasia?

- Can become dysplastic if the agent that caused the metaplasia persists and is capable of inducing dysplasia
- Can be misdiagnosed clinically and perhaps histologically as dysplastic epithelium
- Can be misdiagnosed as carcinoma (such as intestinal metaplasia in the oesophagus)

■ Metastasis

What is the definition of metastasis?

The survival and growth of cells that have migrated or have otherwise been transferred from a malignant tumour to a site or sites distant from the primary.

What are the routes of metastasis? Give examples of tumours that spread in these ways.

- *Lymphatic*: most carcinomas
- *Haematogenous*: most sarcomas, and follicular cell carcinoma of thyroid
- *Transcoelomic*: carcinoma of stomach, colon, pancreas
- *Perineural* (may be in lymphatic channels in the perineurium): adenoid cystic carcinoma of salivary gland
- *CSF*: medulloblastoma, other CNS tumours
- *Iatrogenic*: implantation at surgical operation or as a consequence of one, such as implantation in a granulating area left as the consequence of surgery

Does metastasis from a malignant tumour occur actively or passively?

Actively:

- Detachment of a malignant cell from its neighbours
- Migration through interstitium
- Invasion into a vascular or other space, as above

- Survival in transit
- Invasion of a new endothelium or serosal surface
- Migration into the host tissues
- Development and growth as a metastatic deposit

Do non-malignant cells move into the circulation?

Yes. As well as the cells of the blood:

- Syncytiotrophoblast cells from the fetus' placenta normally invade maternal vessels and may be found in the lungs
- Adrenal cortical cells normally migrate through the wall of the adrenal vein into the blood stream but do not form metastatic deposits

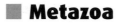 **Metazoa**

What is the definition of a metazoon?

A metazoon is a multicellular organism that has complicated interrelations among its constituent cells with differentiation of cell functions. Even the simplest metazoa have digestive systems. Examples of infective metazoa include helminths (parasitic worms) such as nematodes, cestodes and trematodes. A human being is, strictly speaking, a metazoon.

Why are metazoal infections important?

They enter the differential diagnosis of ophthalmic diseases, neurosurgical diseases, diseases of the gastrointestinal tract, liver and biliary system, and diseases causing lymphoedema that might present surgically.

Which infective metazoa are indigenous to the UK? By what vector or route is the infection acquired?

Toxocara spp.	Nematode	Dogs, cats	Faeco-oral
Enterobius vermicularis	Nematode	Children	Faeco-oral
Echinococcus granulosus	Cestode	Dogs, sheep	Faeco-oral
Taenia saginatum	Cestode	Cattle	Food
Fasciola hepatica	Trematode	Sheep droppings, watercress	Food

Which infective metazoa are not indigenous to the UK but may be acquired by tourists? By what vector or route is the infection acquired?

Ancylosoma duodenale	Nematode	Man	Water-borne
Strongyloides stercoralis	Nematode	Man	Water-borne
Wuchereria bancrofti	Nematode	Mosquito	Bite
Taenia solium	Cestode	Pig	eating infected pork
Schistosoma spp.	Trematode	Man	water-borne from direct penetration of skin
Clonorchis sinensis	Trematode	Man	Eating infected fish

■ Micro-organisms

How do bacteria exert their pathogenic effects?
- Proliferate in the tissues
- Resist phagocytosis in some cases or, if phagocytosed, resist digestion
- Secrete exotoxins when alive, or release endotoxins when dead
- Attach to cell membranes and damage them
- Invade cells and cause tissue damage

What are the body's defences against bacteria?
- Humoral mechanisms
  - Innate
    - Complement activation causing opsonisation and chemotaxis
    - C-reactive protein in pneumococcal infection
      - a globulin made in the liver
      - attaches to C-polysaccharide in the cell wall of pneumococci
  - Acquired
    - Stimulation of antibody production from plasma cells
- Interactive mechanisms
  - Activation of lymphocytes by endotoxins released from organisms
- Cell-mediated
  - Innate
    - Natural killer (NK) cells

- Acquired
  - In relation to bacteria that can grow within human cells, such as mycobacteria and listeria

What are the body's defences against viruses?
- Humoral mechanisms
  - Antibody production
    - Antibodies may bind directly to the virus, may bind to the virus with complement, and may bind to an infected human cell (with or without complement) to cause destruction of the affected cell
- Interferon (IFN) produced by leucocytes and fibroblasts
  - Not specific to particular viruses, and rickettsiae and protozoa can also induce production
  - Effects of IFNs which block translation of viral mRNA in the host cell
    - Inhibit cell division
    - Protect adjacent human cells from infection by a virus
    - Enhance lymphocyte-mediated immune functions
- Cell-mediated
  - NK cells especially in herpesvirus infections
  - Cytokines are released that are chemotactic for macrophages and CD8 killer cells that will destroy the virus-affected cells

What is the difference between a cytokine and a chemokine?

A cytokine is a protein released by a cell that has a specific effect on the interactions between cells or on their behaviour. A chemokine is a type of cytokine that is involved in cell interactions in inflammation.

They are often used interchangably.

■ Multiple endocrine adenopathy

Multiple endocrine disease was first described as multiple endocrine adenomatosis (MEA). It was then realised that, especially in MEA II but also in MEA I, malignant neoplasms could arise or were the rule and so the term was changed to multiple endocrine neoplasia (MEN). The disease of the parathyroid glands in these conditions, however, is usually hyperplasia rather than neoplasia. The term now tends back towards MEA which stands for multiple endocrine adenopathy, a non-committal term that encompasses hyperplasia and neoplasia.

MEA I	
Adenoma or carcinoma of the pancreatic islet cells	Pancreas
Adenoma (very rarely carcinoma) of the pituitary	Pituitary
Hyperplasia of the parathyroid glands	Parathyroids
MEA IIa	
Medullary carcinoma of thyroid	Thyroid
Phaeochromocytoma of adrenal, which may be benign or malignant and has a higher prevalence of bilaterality that in phaeos not related to MEA II	Adrenal
Hyperplasia of the parathyroid glands	Parathyroids
MEA IIb	
Medullary carcinoma of thyroid	Thyroid
Phaeochromocytoma of adrenal, which may be benign or malignant and has a higher prevalence of bilaterality than that of phaeos not related to MEA II	Adrenal
Submucosal neurofibromas of the palate	Palate
Possibly hyperplasia of the parathyroid glands	Parathyroids

■ Mycobacteria

How are mycobacteria classified?

Mycobacteria are beaded bacilli that would be Gram-positive if the stain could penetrate their waxy walls. Ziehl–Neelsen stain is used instead to visualise the organisms which stain pink-red:

- Mycobacteria
  - *Mycobacterium tuberculosis* var. *hominis* and var. *bovis*
  - *Mycobacterium leprae*
- Atypical mycobacteria (those other than the above)
  - *Mycobacterium avium intracellulare*
  - *Mycobacterium marinum*

and also

  - *Mycobacterium ulcerans*
  - *Mycobacterium kansasii*
  - *Mycobacterium smegmatis*
  - *Mycobacterium phlei*

but these are very uncommon

Why are some mycobacteria called "atypical"?

- They have some degree of resistance to the standard antituberculous drugs
- They have different culture characteristics from *Mycobacterium tuberculosis*, such as
  - Pigment production
  - Different rate of growth on culture
  - Different colony appearance

Which mycobacteria are considered atypical and what diseases do they cause?

- *Mycobacterium avium intracellulare*
  - Infections in immunodeficient people such as patients with AIDS
- *Mycobacterium marinum*
  - "Swimming pool granuloma" and skin granulomas in people who keep tropical fish tanks
- *Mycobacterium ulcerans*
  - Buruli ulcer, a spreading subcutaneous infection which causes fat necrosis and lifting of the overlying skin with ulceration
- *Mycobacterium kansasii*
  - Chronic pulmonary infection resembling tuberculosis

What is the histological hallmark of infection with atypical mycobacteria?

- A granuloma which is indistinguishable from a tuberculous granuloma
- In AIDS, non-reactive mycobacterial infection with very numerous organisms and little cellular response

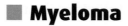

Myeloma

What is myeloma?

- A neoplasm of bone marrow (Gr myelos marrow) composed of a single clone of plasma cells that results in one or more lytic bone lesions in the red marrow and a monotypic globulin in the plasma.
- This can be composed of full immunoglobulin molecules (usually IgG or IgA), free light chains, free heavy chains, or any combination.

Are myelomas always multiple?

- No, though they usually are.
- When proliferating plasma cells form a recognisable mass in tissues other than the marrow it is called a *plasmacytoma*.
- Abnormal plasma cells circulate in patients with myeloma and can be found in microscopic groups in many tissues.

How are the clinical features of myeloma classified?

Related to the local effects of the neoplasm, the effects of the immunoglobulin production and concurrent diseases.

- Local effects
  - Osteolysis
    - Interleukins and tumour necrosis factor α secreted by myeloma cells stimulate osteoclasts to resorb mineralised bone (interleukin 6 is an autocrine growth stimulant for myeloma cells and also inhibits apoptosis)

- The resultant hypercalcaemia causes the complications listed under Hypercalcaemia
  - Pathological fractures
- Direct invasion of structures adjacent to affected bone
  - Extradural spinal cord compression
  - Cranial nerve palsies
- Oversecretion of monotypic immunoglobulin or its components
  - Undersecretion of normal immunoglobulins
    - Susceptibility to infection especially by capsulate organisms
    - pneumonia
    - pyelonephritis
  - Functional abnormalities of B- and T-cells, also contributing to susceptibility to infection
  - Filtration of the protein causes damage to renal tubule epithelial cells
  - Amyloid deposition occurs in many organs but has clinically important effects principally in the renal glomeruli, the heart and the CNS
  - Hyperviscosity syndrome
    - Retinal haemorrhages and other changes
    - Neurological disturbances from thromboses and haemorrhages
    - Excessive bleeding
  - Binding to clotting factor X causing a bleeding diathesis
  - Coating of platelets causing thrombasthenia and a bleeding diathesis

- Coincident diseases
  - Second malignancies, especially of the bowel, breast and bile ducts
  - Unexplained neurological and dermatological changes

How does Waldenström's macroglobulinaemia differ from myeloma?

- Jan Waldenström 1906–96
- Monoclonal proliferation of B-lymphocytes that have not transformed fully into plasma cells
- Characteristically monotypic IgM production
- No focal lytic bone lesions but involvement of the marrow diffusely
- No particular association with amyloidosis
- Anaemia tends to be the predominant feature
  - Depressed haemopoiesis
  - Decreased red cell survival
  - Bleeding tendency and so iron deficiency

■ Necrosis

Define necrosis.

- Necrosis is abnormal tissue death during life. It is energy independent, generally occurs as a result of factors outside the affected cells, and is associated with inflammatory changes.
- (Apoptosis is the degradation of a cell or cells by activation of enzymes present in the cells (i.e. self-digestion) and is an energy-dependent process that does not stimulate an inflammatory response.)
- (A cadaver is neither necrotic nor apoptotic. A cadaver is dead.)

How is necrosis classified?

The three classical types are:

- *Coagulative or structured necrosis*: the tissue architecture is preserved, as seen when a tissue is put into boiling water: the proteins coagulate rapidly from the heat and the architecture is preserved as a consequence. Structured necrosis is seen in kidney, heart and spleen.
- *Colliquative or liquefactive necrosis*: in tissues rich in lipid, lysosomal enzymes denature the fats and cause liquefaction of the affected tissues. Colliquative or liquefactive necrosis is seen in the brain.
- *Caseous or unstructured necrosis*: caseous necrosis is unstructured: wherever it occurs it is impossible to identify the tissue affected by the necrosis as its architecture is

destroyed. It differs histologically from coagulative and colliquative necrosis. Amorphous proteins and degenerate lipid components are present. This type of necrosis is classical for TB.

Give some examples of necrosis in tissues.

- *Fat necrosis*: this can be as a consequence of direct trauma (such as to the female breast) or from enzymatic digestion from pancreatic enzymes released into the serum of a patient with pancreatitis.
- *Wet gangrene*: necrosis in which there is putrefaction cause by infection by anaerobic streptococci, *Bacteroides* spp., *Clostridia* spp.
- *Dry gangrene*: mummification (desiccation) of a tissue without infection such as in an uninfected limb in a diabetic patient.

What does autolysis mean?

Degradation of a cell by activation of enzymes present in the affected cell (i.e. self-digestion) is called *autolysis*. May occur in necrosis or apoptosis but classically occurs post-mortem.

What does heterolysis mean?

Degradation of a cell by activation of enzymes present in cells other than the affected cell (such as digestion of the cell by enzymes from neutrophils, macrophages or perhaps the pancreas) is called *heterolysis*.

Neoplasms

Define *carcinoma* and *sarcoma*.

A *carcinoma* is a malignant tumour of epithelial cells.

A *sarcoma* is a malignant tumour of connective tissue cells.

Can a carcinoma occur in an organ derived from mesoderm?

If the organ contains epithelial cells, yes. Examples include carcinomas of the kidney, ovary, endometrium and fallopian tube.

Other than carcinoma of the skin, what are the four commonest carcinomas in men?

Prostate, bronchopulmonary, colorectal and urinary malignancies.

Is the order the same for the number of deaths caused by the malignancy?

No, changes to bronchopulmonary, prostate, colorectal, urinary malignancy.

And for women?

Commonest are breast, bronchopulmonary, colorectal, uterine malignancies.

Commonest malignant causes of death in order are bronchopulmonary, breast, colorectal, ovarian malignancy.

What histological features do malignant tumours have in common?

- *Mitoses*: increased in number
- *Abnormal mitoses*: tripolar, tetrapolar, sunburst, bizarre
- *Increased N–C ratio*: the nuclear–cytoplasmic ratio changes as the nucleus enlarges
- *Pleomorphism*: variance of size and shape of tumour cells
- *Hyperchromatism*: dark-staining nuclei because of increased amounts of DNA
- *Necrosis*: because of abnormal vascularity
- *Haemorrhage*: because of abnormal vascularity
- *Infiltrative borders*: may be focal or extensive

Which tumours characteristically metastasise to bone?

Tumours of the breast, prostate, bronchus, kidney and thyroid in that order

▓ Nerve injuries

What is the structure of a typical nerve bundle, starting with the innermost aspect?

- The axon, which conducts the impulse
- Around it, Schwann cells wrapped around which make myelin for insulation
- Around a group of axons and Schwann cell membranes, the fibrous endoneurium for continuity; this constitutes a nerve fibre
- Around a group of nerve fibres, the perineurium. The sheath around a group of major nerves (such as mixed motor and sensory bundles) is the epineurium

How are nerve injuries classified in terms of the structure of nerves?

- Neuropraxia:
  - A minor injury to a nerve that can heal with complete recovery of function: the axon is continuous and the damage involves only the myelin sheath to a greater or lesser extent
  - There is no Wallerian degeneration
  - Examples include "pins-and-needles" when there has been minor and temporary nerve compression from crossed legs; "Saturday night paralysis" of the radial nerve by someone sleeping with an arm thrown across a chair back; and temporary paralysis after tourniquet use

- Axonotmesis or axontmesis:
  - Damage to the myelin sheath and axon but with the rest of the nerve structure intact, so there is an intact endoneurial sheath
  - There is Wallerian degeneration distal to the injury
  - The axon will regrow along the sheath if it can
- Neuronotmesis or neurontmesis:
  - Transection of all parts of a nerve or nerve bundle
  - There is Wallerian degeneration distal to the injury
  - Axonal regeneration cannot occur
  - Intraneural fibrosis occurs and blocks axonal regeneration
  - Complete recovery is unlikely but might be improved by careful surgical apposition

(-praxia from Gr ability to do or to perform, with neuro- here replacing a- as in apraxia, loss of the ability to do. -tmesis Gr a cutting also gives us -otomy)

In what ways that are of surgical importance might nerves be damaged?
- Trauma other than bone fracture
  - Relatively common
  - Commonest from aggression: blunt trauma, knives or other penetrating injuries such as from bullets (in most gunshot wounds, a nerve is not divided)
  - Clean accidental lacerations of nerves are rare – injuries from accidental stab wounds and stabs from foreign bodies (shattered glass, falling sheet metal, car crash injuries) might contribute

- Blunt penetrating trauma when the nerves are not cleanly sectioned
- Fractures and fracture–dislocations
  - The probability of nerve injury is doubled with fracture associated with shoulder dislocation
  - Almost all peripheral nerve injuries are associated with a fracture of a bone in the arm or forearm
    - The commonest injury from fracture–dislocation of the elbow is ulnar nerve neurapraxia
    - Radial nerve damage is cause by fracture of the humerus, a common nerve lesion in long bone fracture
- Compartment syndrome injuries
- Stretch injury
  - A nerve can stretch 10–20% before structural damage occurs
  - Typically causes axonotmesis with disruption of axons over long segments of nerve
- Cold injury
  - Frostbite leads to necrosis of all the involved tissues including the peripheral nerves
- Injury to nerves from healing with scar contracture
  - The sciatic nerve can be compressed from scar formation and heterotopic ossification after hip trauma
  - After elbow trauma, scarring can trap the ulnar nerve at the elbow
- Iatrogenic causes
  - Plating of a closed forearm fracture
  - Excessive traction, suture compression, iatrogenic laceration

◼ Nipple discharge

How is nipple discharge defined?

Any cause of leakage of fluid from one or both nipples. About 1 in 20 women referred to a breast clinic have nipple discharge.

Classify nipple discharge.

Different ways:

- Physiological or pathological
- Unilateral or bilateral
- Clear, milky, purulent, bloodstained
- From single or multiple ducts
- Spontaneous flow or only when expressed

List some physiological causes of nipple discharge.

- Neonates: "witches milk" in boys as well as girls
- Pregnancy and lactation
- Mechanical stimulation, especially suckling

List some pathological causes.

- Clear fluid not from the ducts but from the surface of the nipple itself
  - Eczema
  - Paget's disease of nipple
- Milky discharge, galactorrhoea: milk secretion in excess of requirements for breast feeding
  - Mechanical stimulation
  - Hormonal effects at menarche and menopause
  - Stress

- Hyperprolactinaemia
  - Pituitary lactotroph adenoma
  - Hypothalamic overactivity
  - Ectopic prolactin secretion
  - Hypothyroidism
  - Chronic renal failure
  - Iatrogenic: methyldopa, phenothiazines, opiates
- Purulent discharge
  - Bilateral, multiduct: duct ectasia
  - Unilateral, during breast feeding or shortly afterwards: breast abscess
- Bloodstained discharge
  - Unilateral
    - Duct papilloma
    - Intraduct carcinoma
    - Ductal carcinoma
    - Lobular carcinoma
  - Bilateral
    - Bilateral neoplasia

■ Nosocomial infections

What is a nosocomial infection?

An infection acquired specifically as a consequence of being in hospital (Gr *nosocomium* hospital).

That is, not a cold virus or influenza which happens to be acquired in hospital that could have been acquired anywhere, but an infection that is unusual in the general population and is considered to be acquired as a direct consequence of a hospital stay.

What are the commonest types of nosocomial infection?

- Urinary tract infections
- Surgical wound infections
- Skin and spreading soft tissue infections
- Pneumonia
- Bacteraemia

What patients are at most risk of a nosocomial infection?

- Patients with AIDS, other immunocompromised states, prostheses
- Patients in intensive care units
- Patients on surgical wards
- Patients, especially children with leukaemia, on paediatric wards who acquire measles or chicken pox
- Patients with urinary or intravenous catheters on any ward
- Patients receiving long-term antibiotics

- Patients on wards that have an outbreak of antibiotic resistant infection such as methicillin-resistant *Staphylococcus aureus* (MRSA)

What are the sources of infection?
- People
  - Incidental carriers
- Fomites (anything inanimate that comes into contact with a patient) (Latin *fomes = tinder* in the pleural makes *fomites*. The modern singular of fomites, *fomite*, is a back formation)
  - Surgical instruments
  - Anaesthetic equipment
  - Humidifiers
- Parenteral fluids
- Operating theatres

What are the routes of infection?
- Direct contact
  - People
  - Fomites
- Airborne
  - Droplet spread
    - Sneezing and other nasal spread
    - Aerosol spread from humidifiers, nebulisers, ventilation systems
  - Dust spread
- Ingestion
  - Food poisoning

■ Oedema, transudate and exudate

What is oedema?

An abnormal accumulation of fluid in intercellular spaces. This may be the result of a transudate or an exudate into the connective tissues and may be local or generalised.

What is a transudate?

A transudate is characteristically formed by an imbalance between the hydrostatic pressures and oncotic pressures, resulting in a fluid of low protein content traversing an intact endothelial surface. A transudate characteristically has a protein content of <30 g/l and a specific gravity of <1.020.

What is an exudate?

An exudate is characteristically formed by an inflammatory process resulting in a fluid of high protein content traversing a damaged endothelial surface. An exudate characteristically has a protein content of >30 g/l and a specific gravity of >1.020.

Under what circumstances does a transudate occur?

- Factors governing the amount of extracellular fluid
  - ■ The pressure of blood in the capillaries
  - ■ The oncotic pressure of the plasma
  - ■ The pressure in the tissues around the capillaries and the capacity to drain lymph from them

- Factors that raise capillary pressure
  - Congestive cardiac failure
  - Fluid retention because of salt retention
  - Fluid retention because of renal failure
  - Local events such as venous thrombosis
- Factors that lower oncotic pressure
  - Low plasma proteins because of deficient formation such as hepatic failure, malnutrition
  - Low plasma proteins because of protein loss such as from nephrotic syndrome and severe burns
- Causes of lymphoedema
  - Filariasis
  - Irradiation
  - Regional lymphadenectomy

How do you classify an exudate in terms of its content or formation and in terms of its causative disease?

- Serous
  - In pleural, pericardial and peritoneal cavities such as in malignant ascites, pleurisy
- Haemorrhagic
  - In TB pleurisy, peritonitis
- Purulent
  - In *Escherichia coli* peritonitis
- Fibrinous
  - In pericarditis
- Pseudomembranous (used to be called catarrhal)
  - In Corynebacterial infections
  - Results of *Clostridium difficile* toxin
- More than one of the above

■ Organisation, granulation tissue and wound healing

What do we mean by organisation?

The transformation of inanimate material such as clot, thrombus or pus into living tissue responsive to the growth control factors of the body by replacement by granulation tissue.

What is granulation tissue?

Granulation tissue is composed of proliferating capillary buds, fibroblasts and macrophages. It is a characteristic part of healing by second intention but can sometimes have deleterious consequences, such as joint destruction in rheumatoid arthritis (RA) by granulation tissue (called *pannus* historically and for no good reason nowadays).

Is granulation tissue resistant to damage by physical trauma, chemical agents, ionising radiation and infection?

- Physical trauma: no
- Chemical agents: no
- Ionising radiation: no
- Infection: yes, almost as good as in intact epithelium

■ Osteoarthritis

What is osteoarthritis (OA)?

A common degenerative joint disease that involves synovial joints only with recurrent or abnormal load-bearing on normal cartilage or normal load-bearing on weakened cartilage, or both.

How is OA classified?

Into primary, secondary and generalised OA:

- Primary OA
  - Unknown aetiology
  - 15% of the adult population in the UK
  - No known cause, though associations include
    - Obesity
    - Familial association
    - Sex: female > male in polyarticular OA
    - Joint shape and tendency to suffer mechanical damage
- Secondary OA, secondary to
  - RA
  - Misaligned and non-aligned fractures
    - Fracture through a joint space
    - Misalignment after fracture
    - Direct joint trauma
  - Occupational trauma such as repetitive strain
  - Gout
  - Pseudogout (pyrophosphate arthropathy)
  - Paget's disease of bone

- Avascular necrosis of the femoral head
- Osteochondritis
- Neuropathic arthritis
- Inflammatory joint disease
  - Infective arthritis: gonococcus, salmonella
  - Non-infective inflammatory arthritides other than RA
    - Ankylosing spondylitis
    - Psoriatic arthropathies
- Congenital causes
  - Achondroplasia
  - Congenital causes of fracture such as abnormal fragility of bone
- Caisson disease
- Generalised OA
  - Associated with human leucocyte antigen (HLA) A1 and B8
  - Immune complexes found in the synovium and cartilage
  - Rheumatoid factor more prevalent than in other types of OA

What joints are affected in OA?

OA involves synovial joints only:

- Hip joint
- Knee joint
- Shoulder joint

- Elbow joint
- Interphalangeal joint
- Temporomandibular joint and apparatus
- Joints between the ossicles in the middle ear
- Facet joints in the vertebral column

■ Osteomyelitis

What is the definition of osteomyelitis?
Inflammation of the bone and bone marrow

How are the causes of osteomyelitis classified?
- Infective causes
  - *Staphylococcus aureus*
  - *Escherichia coli*
  - *Streptococcus* spp.
  - Other bowel organisms such as *Pseudomonas* spp.
  - *Salmonella* spp. in patients with sickle cell disease
  - Viruses
  - Fungi
  - Parasites
- Non-infective causes
  - Radiotherapy

What are the classical pathological sequelae of osteomyelitis in a long bone such as the tibia?
- Suppuration with pus in the marrow cavity
- Sequestrum: the dead (and sometimes living) bone within the periosteum that forms the inner part of the infected bone and marrow
- Involucrum: the reaction of the periosteum to form new bone that envelops the infected site and contains it
- Cloacae: holes in the involucrum through which pus formed in the medulla discharges (L. *cloaca*, a sewer)

- Sinus: the track that forms for drainage from the cloacae to the skin
- Septicaemia, pyaemia

What are the late complications of osteomyelitis?
- Amyloidosis
- Malignant change in the sinus – Marjolin's ulcer, a squamous cell carcinoma in the sinus track (*not* malignant change in a venous ulcer)
- Septicaemia, pyaemia
- Suppurative arthritis

■ Osteoporosis

What is osteoporosis?
A reduction in the total mass of normally mineralised bone.

How is osteoporosis classified?
Into local and generalised, and the latter into menopause-related, age-related and secondary.

What causes of localised osteoporosis are there?
These include:
- Fracture: the fracture ends develop local osteoporosis
- Metastatic carcinoma: osteoporosis develops at the site of the metastasis
- Radiotherapy
- Thalassaemia
- Immobilisation of a limb or part of a limb

What are the features of menopause-related generalised osteoporosis?
- Bone formation is:
  - Faster than resorption until about 30 years
  - In equilibrium with resorption at 30 years
  - Slower than resorption after 30 years
- Bone loss is fastest in the first few years after menopause
- Rate of bone loss slows after that but loss persists into the postmenopausal years:
  - Trabecular bone is lost quicker than cortical bone
  - Osteoclasts increase in number and form larger resorption lacunae

What are the features of age-related generalised osteoporosis?

- Both sexes lose bone over a lifetime
- Women lose about half of trabecular bone mass, men lose one-third
- Osteoblasts fail to fill resorption lacunae adequately with new bone

What are the risk factors for generalised osteoporosis?

- Sex: women have less bone to start with, and lose bone more rapidly because of the menopause
- Body size: small, thin-boned women are more at risk
- Age: the greater the age, the greater the risk in both sexes
- Family history
- Ethnic origin: caucasian and Asian women are more affected than Black and Latino women
- Low sex hormone concentrations in both sexes
- Iatrogenic: glucocorticoids and some anticonvulsants
- Inactive lifestyle or extended bed rest
- A lifetime diet low in calcium and vitamin D
- Smoking
- Excessive alcohol

What are the causes of secondary osteoporosis?

Osteoporosis arises secondary to:

- Hypogonadism in either sex
- Cushing's syndrome from any cause, including iatrogenic
- Acromegaly
- Hyperthyroidism

Osteosarcoma and chondrosarcoma

What is an osteosarcoma?

A tumour arising from a primitive mesenchymal bone-forming cell characterised by production of osteoid and the bone isoenzyme of alkaline phosphatase:

- A rare neoplasm, affecting
  - Children and young adults, age range: 10–25 years
  - Blacks slightly more than Whites
  - Men more than women
  - People with Paget's disease, though the apparent risk tends to be exaggerated
- Arises most commonly in long bones
  - Femur (40%, most near the knee)
  - Tibia (20%, most near the knee)
  - Humerus (10%, most near the shoulder)

What are the risk factors for osteosarcoma?

The cause is unknown in most cases. Risk factors include:

- Rapid bone growth
  - Increased incidence during adolescent growth
  - High incidence in large dogs
  - Typical location near the metaphyseal growth plate of long bones
- Exposure to radiation, especially particulate radiation from isotopes such as radioactive strontium that are taken up by bone

- Genetic predisposition
  - Retinoblastoma is associated with a particularly high risk of osteosarcoma development
  - Hereditary multiple exostoses
- Pre-existing bone disease, rarely
  - Paget's disease
  - Fibrous dysplasia
  - Enchondromatosis
- Li–Fraumeni syndrome

What is a chondrosarcoma?

A tumour arising from a primitive mesenchymal cartilage-forming cell characterised by tumour matrix formation that is entirely chondroid. *Any* bone formation in what is otherwise a chondrosarcoma makes it an osteosarcoma.

- A rare neoplasm, affecting
  - Adults over the age of 35 years
  - Children very rarely
  - The elderly: the incidence increases with age (starting at 35 years)
  - Men slightly more than women
  - Blacks and Whites equally
  - People with Ollier's disease, Maffucci's syndrome, chondromatosis
- Arises most commonly in the axial skeleton
  - Pelvic bones, especially the ilium
  - Ribs, scapulae, sternum
  - Vertebral bodies
- Appendicular chondrosarcoma usually arises in a chondroma or ecchondroma

■ **p53**

Name a growth suppressor gene and describe its action.

p53 is one of the commonest growth inhibitor genes to become abnormal in human cancer.

DNA damage in a cell results in activation of *p53* gene to make p53 protein. This arrests the cell cycle by increasing the concentration of the cyclin-dependent kinase inhibitor p21 protein and so prevents the damaged DNA being replicated. The p53 protein will force the cell into apoptosis if the DNA defect is not remedied. Abnormalities of the *p53* gene prevent this protective mechanism.

By what mechanisms does p53 function become diminished?

- Mutation of the *p53* gene
- Binding of anti-p53 protein to p53 protein. Normally p53 is regulated by the growth promoter *mdm-2*. Overactivity of *mdm-2* results in excess protein product which binds with and inactivates p53 protein
- Metabolism of p53 protein by viruses such as human papilloma virus (HPV)
- Abnormal handling of p53 protein in the cytoplasm so that it becomes inaccessible and so effectively inactive

What other growth suppressor genes are important surgically?

- Retinoblastoma gene: in retinoblastoma and osteosarcoma
- APC gene: in familial adenomatous polyposis
- Wilms' tumour gene: in nephroblastoma
- BRCA1, BRCA2: in breast and ovarian carcinoma

▉ Paget's diseases

What diseases or other medical entities are named for Sir James Paget (1814–1895)?

- Paget's disease of bone
- Paget's disease of nipple
- Paget's disease of penis and scrotum (described before the vulval disease)
- Paget's disease of vulva
- Paget's disease of the perineum, axilla, eyelid and external ear (in decreasing prevalence)
- Paget's abscess
- Paget–von Schrötter disease
- Paget's sign

Paget was the first to recognise trichinosis in muscle, but there was no eponymous attachment.

What is Paget's disease of extramammary skin?

Paget's disease of the vulva, perineum, penis, scrotum, axilla, eyelid and external ear has features in common with Paget's disease of the nipple but does not have the same connotations of an obligatory underlying neoplasm:

- Relatively common in elderly White women and less commonly White men, rare in Blacks of both sexes
- Differential diagnosis includes Bowen's disease, superficial spreading melanoma in situ, eczema, psoriasis and fungal infection

- Two main origins of the Pagetic cells:
  - In the epidermis with spread along the epidermis to involve sweat ducts and glands, and occasionally into the dermis
  - In an underlying adenocarcinoma in the gastrointestinal or genitourinary system with spread into the epidermis
- Associated with an underlying malignancy in only about 50% of cases (an even smaller percentage in the vulva according to many reports) unlike mammary Paget's disease.

What was a Paget's abscess?

An abscess that forms around the residue of a former abscess after its apparent cure.

What was Paget–von Schrötter disease?

Primary thrombosis of the axillary vein and associated radicles associated sometimes with severe physical exercise but sometimes with no apparent predisposing event.

What was Paget's sign?

A clinical test for fluctuation in a skin mass by using two fingers pressing on the mass and moving apart, while a third finger palpates the centre of the mass. All three fingers detect the presence of fluid in the mass by the transmission of pressure from the central finger to the other two.

Pancreatitis I: classification and pathogenesis

Why is acute pancreatitis of surgical importance?

- Pancreatitis is important in the differential diagnosis of acute abdominal pain
- The morbidity and mortality of patients with pancreatitis are significantly increased if they are subjected to inappropriate laparotomy (cholecystectomy as the treatment for the primary cause of the pancreatitis needs careful timing)
- A surgeon may be required to manage a patient with pancreatitis, at least as an emergency admission
- A surgeon may cause pancreatitis

How would you classify the pathogenetic mechanisms that result in acute pancreatitis?

These can be classified as aetiological agents that affect:

- Duct-drainage system
- Pancreatic acinar cells directly
- Blood supply

Some agents such as alcohol and radiotherapy can do all three.

What is the pathogenesis of acute pancreatitis?

- Local
    - Chemical destruction of pancreatic exocrine cells leading to:
        - Release of lytic enzymes which destroy more pancreatic exocrine cells

- Acute oedema
- Haemorrhage into the pancreas owing to destruction of blood vessels by amylase, lipase and proteases
- Secondary peritonitis
- Systemic
  - Inflammatory mediators

What are the complications of acute pancreatitis?
- Pancreatic abscess
- Pancreatic pseudocyst
- Severe destructive pancreatic haemorrhage
- Duodenal obstruction
- Chylous ascites
- Misdiagnosis as perforated viscus with consequent morbidity

What criteria are used for assessing acute pancreatitis clinically?
- Acute physiology and chronic health evaluation score (APACHE III)
- Ranson criteria
- Glasgow score

Pancreatitis II: acute pancreatitis

Give some aetiologies of acute pancreatitis.

- Alcohol
  - Change of tone in the sphincter of Oddi permitting bile reflux into the pancreatic duct
  - Direct cytotoxic effect on acinar cells in the pancreas
  - Related to hypotension and hypothermia
  - Physical trauma with disruption
- Gallstones
  - Blocking the ampulla of Vater permitting reflux of bile into the pancreatic duct
  - Even when the ductal systems are separate, fibrosis as the result of a stone in the common bile duct can distort the adjacent pancreatic duct by contraction
- Trauma
  - Car crash, train crash
  - Other direct abdominal trauma such as playing rugby
- Metabolic abnormalities
  - Hypercalcaemia
  - Hypercholesterolaemia
  - Hypercortisolaemia
- Iatrogenic causes
  - Direct trauma from operative surgery to the upper abdomen
  - Ischaemia from ligation of the pancreaticoduodenal artery

- Drugs: thiazides, furosemide, steroids, morphine
- Cytotoxic drugs
- Radiotherapy
- Endoscopic retrograde cholangiopancreatography (ERCP)
- Viruses
  - Mumps
  - Coxsackie B
- Congenital causes
  - Cystic fibrosis
  - Haemochromatosis
  - Cysts of the pancreatic and biliary ducts

■ Paperwork

What information is needed on a request form accompanying a specimen to pathology?

- At least, the minimum data set for patient identification
  - Varies in different hospitals
  - Always has the patient's name, registry number or equivalent
  - The age of the patient
  - Where relevant, the sex of the patient if not already apparent (first names like Alex, Nicky, Hilary and Kim could be used by either sex)
- Name of the consultant who has admitted the patient
- Referring doctor's name and contact number (pager or mobile)
- Clinical details relevant to the case
- Reason for the request
  - This could be implicit when the clinical details are, for example, carcinoma of transverse colon or lump in breast
  - Specific questions for the pathologist to address that would not form part of his or her routine reporting set (such as response to treatment, reason for circulating eosinophilia or involvement of nerve bundles)
  - Any confounding variables that are important in the assessment of the case (such as congenital adrenal hyperplasia in a patient with an enlarged testis, or previous treatment of an unusual skin rash with high-dose steroids before the biopsy specimen was taken)

- Any special requirements
  - Specimen photography
  - Photomicrography as a print for the notes or as a slide for lectures
  - Retention of the specimen
    - for collection by the patient
    - for legal reasons

What happens to the forms and specimens in the histopathology laboratory?

- Retention indefinitely of all
  - Request forms
  - Slides
  - Blocks
  - Laboratory copies of reports
- Retention, usually for 6 weeks, of the specimen remaining after the blocks have been taken
- Issuing to the referring doctor of the ward copy of the report form

What would be a minimum data set for a specimen with carcinoma?

- Macroscopic part of the report
  - Site of the tumour
  - Size of the tumour
  - Appearance of the tumour, whether it is ulcerated, haemorrhagic or necrotic
  - How the tumour is behaving macroscopically
    - Tissues involved by direct spread

- Involvement of vital structures
- Involvement of local and sentinel lymph nodes
  - Whether the tumour appears excised macroscopically
- Microscopic part of the report
  - Tumour site
  - Tumour type (such as squamous cell carcinoma, adenocarcinoma, transitional cell carcinoma, carcinosarcoma)
  - Differentiation or grade of the tumour (well, moderately or poorly differentiated, or undifferentiated)
    - Any specific grading schemes used, such as Gleason grading of prostatic adenocarcinoma
  - The tissues involved directly by the tumour
    - Involvement of different levels of the bowel or skin
    - Involvement of the nipple
    - Vascular space invasion
    - Tumour present of the serosa of the specimen
  - The tissues involved by metastases of the tumour that might be in the specimen
    - Local and distant lymph nodes by metastatic spread, with specific mention of the sentinel node when relevant
    - The ovaries by transcoelomic spread
  - The TNM stage or the Dukes' stage or whatever relevant staging is used, or information sufficient for the stage to be worked out
  - A comment when a specific question has been asked by the referring ward clinicians
  - A conclusion when the case is long and complicated (some pathologists dislike conclusions as they fear that these are the only parts of the reports that will be read)

■ Paraneoplastic syndromes

What is the definition of a paraneoplastic syndrome?

A paraneoplastic syndrome is one in which there are symptoms and signs as a result of a neoplasm *other than* by its direct involvement, metastatic spread or associated cachexia and which cannot be explained by secretion of hormones or enzymes eutopic to the tumour.

Syndromes caused by a neoplasm by direct involvement, metastatic spread, cachexia or eutopic hormone secretion would be called *neoplastic syndromes.*

Why is a knowledge of paraneoplastic syndromes surgically important?

Because the symptoms and signs:

- May be the earliest clinical manifestation of a neoplasm
- Can lead to morbidity or death
- Can mimic other diseases and divert attention from the underlying neoplasm
- Can mimic metastatic neoplasia, leading to up-staging of the neoplasm

How are paraneoplastic syndromes classified?

- Endocrine
    - Cushing's syndrome: ectopic adrenocorticotropic hormone (ACTH) or similar polypeptide
    - Antidiuretic hormone (ADH) secretion: ectopic ADH or similar polypeptide
    - Hypercalcaemia: parathyroid hormone-related protein (PTHrp), vitamin D activation

- Haematological
  - Polycythaemia
  - Disseminated intravascular coagulopathy
  - Thrombocythaemia
  - Thrombotic tendency, sometimes classical thrombophlebitis migrans
  - Non-infective thrombotic endocarditis
- Dermatological and soft tissue diseases
  - Acanthosis nigricans
  - Dermatomyositis
  - Erythema gyratum repens
  - Erythrodermia
  - Clubbing of digits
- Neuromuscular
  - Polymyositis
  - Myopathies with or without frank myasthenia
  - Cerebellar degeneration
  - Demyelinating disorders

Which neoplasms are classically associated with paraneoplastic syndromes?

- Bronchial carcinoma (especially oat cell and squamous cell carcinoma) causing Eaton–Lambert syndrome, myopathy and hypercalcaemia
- Breast carcinoma causing hypercalcaemia
- Pancreatic adenocarcinoma causing thrombophlebitis migrans

■ Pathological fractures

What is the definition of a pathological fracture?

A fracture through a previously abnormal bone – one that has existing disease – irrespective of the force of the physical trauma.

What are the causes of pathological fracture?

- Osteoporosis
- Metastatic carcinoma (osteolytic and osteosclerotic metastases both predispose to pathological fracture)
- Metabolic bone disease
  - Rickets with greenstick fractures
  - Osteomalacia
  - Renal bone disease
  - "Brown tumour" of hyperparathyroidism
- Primary neoplasia
- Congenital: osteogenesis imperfecta
- Paget's disease of bone
- Iatrogenic
  - Treatment with steroids
  - Radiotherapy causing bone necrosis

▪ Platelets

What are platelets?

Cytoplasmic fragments of megakaryocytes that release clotting, vasoactive and other substances locally to manage a breach in an endothelial cell surface.

How are platelets formed?

- Cytoplasmic fragments of megakaryocytes
  - Megakaryocytes mature by nuclear division without cell division (*endomitosis*)
  - Their cytoplasm demarcates into platelet subunits which are released into the circulation by megakaryocyte fragmentation
- No nucleus and so no continuous ability to synthesise enzymes
- Regulated to meet the demand for circulating platelets by growth factors such as thrombopoietin

What is the structure of a platelet?

- Its cell membrane has:
  - Reactive proteins that attach to:
    - von Willebrand factor (vWF)
    - Fibrinogen
- Its cytoplasm contains:
  - Actin and myosin fibres that control its shape

- Storage granules
  - *Alpha granules*: clotting factors V, VIII, fibrinogen and vWF, platelet factor IV (a heparin antagonist) and platelet-derived growth factor
  - *Dense granules*: 5-HT, ADP, catecholamines, calcium
  - *Glycogen granules*: provide the energy source for platelet reactions
- Thromboxane and prostaglandins

How are platelet numbers controlled?

- The normal is about 150–400 $\times$ 10^9/l of blood
- They have a life span of 7–10 days
- They are mostly in the general circulation:
  - Two-thirds of platelets from the bone marrow stay in the circulation
  - One third are in a pool in the spleen that exchanges with circulating platelets
- The number is affected by splenomegaly, which sequesters more platelets but does not intrinsically lead to a shortened platelet survival

What happens when a platelet encounters a breach in an endothelial surface?

There is:

- Adhesion to exposed collagen by platelet membrane proteins and vWF, a very large molecule that bridges the gaps between platelets and between platelets and collagen

- Change of shape from a disc to a sphere by rearrangement of microtubules
- Release of granule contents: ADP, 5-HT, catecholamine, calcium
- Binding of fibrinogen to circulating platelets nearby to polymerise to fibrin and fill the gaps (stimulated by ADP)
- Binding of other clotting factors to the platelet surface, including factors V and VIII
- Consolidation of the platelet plug by thromboxane and prostaglandin
- Clot retraction when platelets trapped in the clot extend pseudopodia that attach to pseudopodia on adjacent platelets and, over time, contract

Why does aspirin prevent coagulation?

- Aspirin interfers with cyclo-oxygenase (COX) enzymes necessary for the formation of thromboxane and prostaglandin in platelets and endothelial cells
- The block in the platelet is permanent as it does not have a nucleus that would support regeneration of more COX
- The effect of the aspirin decreases over a week as new platelets replace those exposed to aspirin
- In endothelial cells, the block is not permanent: COX is regenerated as endothelial cells have nuclei

How do patients with thrombocytopaenia present?

- Petechiae and ecchymoses
- Epistaxis
- Bleeding from gums

- Melaena
- Menorrhagia
- Retinal haemorrhages
- Splenomegaly

How do patients with thrombocytosis present?

- Splenomegaly
- Haemorrhages
- Thrombotic episodes
  - Digital ischaemia
  - Coronary thrombosis

Polycythaemia

How is polycythaemia classified?

Primary, secondary and relative. In primary polycythaemia, the erythropoietin concentration is normal.

What type of disease is primary polycythaemia?

Polycythaemia vera, one of the myeloproliferative diseases. The others include myelofibrosis, chronic myeloid leukaemia and essential thrombocythaemia.

How is secondary polycythaemia classified?

- Causes due to appropriate erythropoietin excess:
  - Emphysema
  - Congestive cardiac failure
  - Haemoglobinopathies: high-affinity haemoglobin Chesapeake Bay
- Causes due to inappropriate erythropoietin excess, such as:
  - Renal neoplasms
  - Cerebellar haemangioblastoma
  - Phaeochromocytoma
  - Hepatocellular carcinoma
  - Prostatic adenocarcinoma
  - Uterine leiomyoma

What does relative polycythaemia mean?

Apparent polycythaemia because of a reduction in plasma volume.

Stress polycythaemia results from contraction of extracellular fluid volume characteristically in middle-aged businessmen.

■ Polyps of the large bowel

On what general pathology principles are polyps of the large bowel classified?

- Metaplastic or hyperplastic: by far the commonest
- Inflammatory
  - So-called benign lymphoid polyp
  - Polyps in ulcerative colitis and rarely Crohn's disease
  - Infective polyps: schistosomal & amoebic polyps
- Hamartomatous
  - Peutz–Jeghers' polyps
  - Juvenile polyps
- Neoplastic
  - Tubular adenoma
  - Tubulovillous papilloma
  - Villous papilloma

What are the complications of large bowel neoplastic polyps?

- Malignant change
- Ulceration and blood loss leading to iron deficiency anaemia
- Infection
- Intussusception
- Protein loss
- Potassium loss

What syndromes are associated with polyps of the large bowel?

- Peutz–Jeghers' syndrome
- Familial adenomatous polyposis
- Acromegaly

Prostate cancer

What is the commonest type of carcinoma of the prostate?

Adenocarcinoma characteristically arising in the posterolateral aspects of the gland. Occasionally, the tumour has foci of squamous differentiation.

What are the predisposing factors to carcinoma of the prostate?

The aetiology of carcinoma of the prostate is unknown but there are related features that might have a bearing in a particular case.

- The incidence is low in
  - Eunuchs
  - Men with Kleinfelter's syndrome
  - Men with a high serum oestrogen concentration, such as may be associated with cirrhosis of the liver
- Orchiectomy causes slowing of growth and in some cases regression
- Testosterone stimulates tumour growth (there is no evidence to date that testosterone causes prostatic cancer)

How is prostatic carcinoma diagnosed clinically?

- On trans-urethral resection of the prostate (TURP)
- On core biopsy taken per rectum
- On retropubic prostatectomy specimens

- By cytology on expressed prostatic secretions, very rarely
- Serologically (and presumptively) by raised tumour markers prostate specific antigen (PSA) and prostate specific acid phosphatase

What grading system is often used for carcinoma of the prostate?

Gleason grading, based on the histological pattern of growth. The scoring takes into account two aspects:

- The degree of glandular differentiation
- The growth pattern of invasion

The most predominant and the next most predominant aspects of growth are examined and scored. In an otherwise well differentiated tumour, there may be tiny areas of very poorly differentiated adenocarcinoma and these are ignored if they do not represent the most and next-most predominant aspect.

Each aspect is scored 1–5, where 1 is a very well differentiated tumour and/or a localised tumour or both, and 5 is a very poorly differentiated and/or widely infiltrating tumour or both. The scores for the area under examination are added to give a final score out of 10. The tumour will behave, it is assumed from this grading, according to the mean of the two final scores (rather than according to the worse score, which seems paradoxical).

Tumours with a score of 2 (i.e. 1 + 1, the lowest possible) have a very good prognosis with a very low death rate. Tumours with an average score of 9 have a higher death rate of 0.2 deaths per patient-year.

How is carcinoma of the prostate staged?

- By TNM usually
- A clinical system is in use in the USA:
  - A: clinically silent
  - B: palpable on rectal examination
  - C: spread through the prostatic capsule
  - D: metastatic spread

What are the characteristic routes of spread of prostatic carcinoma?

- Local direct spread into adjacent prostate
- Through the prostatic capsule into adjacent tissues
  - Commonly into prostatic urethra, seminal vesicles, bladder base, adjacent adipose tissues
  - Rarely into rectum
- Lymphatic spread to
  - Periprostatic local lymph nodes
  - Pelvic nodes
  - Para-aortic nodes
  - Lymph nodes in the thorax and elsewhere
- Haematogenous spread to
  - Bone, especially pelvis and lumbar spine, with osteosclerotic deposits
    - Systemic venous spread with dissemination
    - Retrograde spread through the prostatic venous plexus of Batson to the vertebral veins

■ Protein electrophoresis

What is the difference between plasma and serum?
Plasma contains all of the constituent proteins of the circulation.

Serum is the same but deficient in clotting factors.

What do the globulin peaks on an electrophoretic separation of serum proteins represent?
- α1 band: α1-antitrypsin (protease inhibitor), high-density lipoprotein
- α2 band: α2 macroglobulin, haptoglobin
- β1 and β2 band: low-density lipoprotein, transferrin
- β2 band: β2 microglobulin
- γ band: immunoglobulins

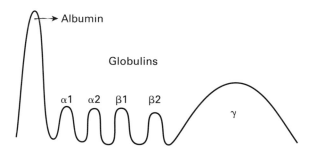

Why is serum used for electrophoresis rather than plasma?
As fibrinogen would swamp over the α and β peaks due to polymerisation.

What is the function of α1-antitrypsin?

- A better term is protease inhibitor, as α1-antitrypsin acts against many lytic enzymes, most specifically against macrophage-derived elastases
- Patients with deficiency tendency to develop emphysema, hepatitis and cirrhosis

■ *Proteus* infection

What species of *Proteus* are of clinical importance?
Proteus vulgaris and *Proteus mirabilis*.

What types of infection are typically caused by *Proteus* spp.?
Urinary tract infections.

What effects on the chemical constituents of urine does a urinary tract infection by *Proteus* spp. have?
The urease from *Proteus* splits urea into ammonium groups and carbonate groups. The pH of the urine rises.

So why does not ammonium carbonate form without any effect on pH?
All tissues of the body are permeable to carbonate and so this can diffuse away, leaving the ammonium radicals which make the urine alkaline.

What effect does this have?
There is an increased proclivity for deposition of calcium salts, with the formation of staghorn calculi and other stones.

What complications follow alkalinisation of urine?
Renal calculi, especially calcium ammonium carbonate staghorn calculi which are predisposed to form in an alkaline medium.

What is important about the growth of *Proteus* spp. on a culture plate?

Proteus does not form colonies. It swarms aggressively all over the culture plate. If the mid-stream urine specimen is not received in the microbiology laboratory promptly, *Proteus* can overgrow other organisms by swarming. When a mixed infection is suspected, a specific culture medium to suppress swarming is used such as CLED medium (which contains cysteine and lactulose and is electrolyte-deficient).

Proto-oncogenes and oncogenes

What is an oncogene?

Genes were discovered in tumour cells that stimulated their proliferation and so were called oncogenes. Other genes were found that suppressed tumour cell growth. Later it was established that both of these gene types in their unmutated or unstimulated forms were found in all normal cells. These forms were called proto-oncogenes. They have an effect on cell proliferation by stimulation and inhibition of growth.

Proto-oncogenes are divided into growth promoter genes (normal, unmutated oncogenes) and growth inhibitor genes (so-called "*tumour suppressor genes*" which suppress growth of all cells and not just tumours).

How do proto-oncogenes become activated into abnormal modulators of cell proliferation?

- *Amplification*: increased copies of the proto-oncogene result in excessive activity
- *Point mutation*: conversion of a proto-oncogene into a permanently active gene
- *Incorporation of a new promoter*: viruses can insert promoter sequences into human DNA and, depending on the site, can activate proto-oncogenes
- *Incorporation of enhancer sequences*: viruses can insert enhancer sequences into human DNA and have an effect similar to promoter insertion

- *Translocation of chromosomal material*: abnormal activation of proto-oncogenes can result from translocation of the chromosomal material bearing the code for the proto-oncogene onto another chromosome on which there is an active enhancer or promoter site that affects the proto-oncogene

How do oncogenes and their products act?

- On signal transduction pathways (such as *ras* and *abl*)
- On regulation of nuclear activity (such as *myc*)
- On growth factors and their receptors (such as *sis*, *erb*B-1 and *erb*B-2)
- On inhibition of apoptosis (such as *bcl*-2)

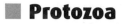

Protozoa

What is a protozoon?
A protozoon is a single-celled, nucleate organism that possesses all processes necessary for reproduction.

Why are protozoal infections clinically important?
Because protozoa enter the differential diagnosis of ophthalmic diseases, neurosurgical diseases, diseases of the gastrointestinal tract and diseases causing splenomegaly that might present surgically.

Give examples of infective protozoa that are indigenous to the UK. By what vector or route is the infection acquired?
- *Toxoplasma gondii*
  - Ophthalmic complications
    - Kitten faeces (adult cats are almost all immune)
    - Dog faeces
    - Eating infected meat
- *Trichomonas vaginalis*
  - Vaginal infection as a sexually transmitted disease
- *Giardia lamblia*
  - Enteritis
    - Contaminated water (rare in UK)
- *Cryptosporidium* spp.
  - Enteritis
    - Animal transmission, transmission from human sewage

Give examples of infective protozoa that are not indigenous to the UK but may be acquired by travellers. By what vector or route is the infection acquired?

- *Entamoeba histolytica*: contaminated water
- *Giardia lamblia*: contaminated water
- Trypanosomiasis: bites from several insect species, including tsetse fly
- Leishmaniasis: sand fly bite

■ Pyogenic granuloma

What is a pyogenic granuloma?

An overgrowth of proliferating capillaries in excess of the body's needs. Macrophages and fibroblasts may be present but are not considered to be part of the lesion. A plasma cell infiltrate is often present.

A pyogenic granuloma is:

- Not intrinsically pyogenic: pus may form because of infection if the lesion ulcerates but is absent otherwise
- Not a granuloma

What are the clinical features of a pyogenic granuloma?

- Arises on digits, earlobes, occasionally surgical wounds
- Develops rapidly, usually at a site of injury but not always
- Bleeds easily on light trauma
- Is either white from hyperkeratosis of the intact overlying epidermis, or red when ulcerated because of the blood flowing through the component capillaries
- Occasionally resolves spontaneously but usually requires intervention

What is the differential diagnosis?

- Amelanotic melanoma
- Squamous cell carcinoma
- Paronychia

- Viral wart
- Molluscum contagiosum

How is pyogenic granuloma managed?
- Surgical excision
- Cryotherapy
- Cautery

▮ Resolution and repair

What is meant by resolution and repair?
- Resolution
  - Replacement of damaged tissue by fully functional tissue normally found at that site (with the implication that no scar tissue forms in pure resolution)
  - Found in healing of defects of the liver and bone marrow and of mucosal defects of the alimentary and urinary tracts
- Repair
  - Replacement of damaged tissue by fibrosis or gliosis which fills or bridges the defect but has no intrinsic specialised function relevant to the organ in which repair occurs
  - Found in most instances of inflammatory or other damage to tissues, either alone or in combination with some degree of resolution

What is an erosion?
A partial loss of an epithelial or mucosal surface which heals by resolution.

What is an ulcer?
A full-thickness loss of epithelium or mucosa which heals by repair with or without some degree of resolution.

What factors influence the rate of healing of an ulcer?
- Local
  - Ischaemia
  - Hypostasis

- Anaesthesia and hypoaesthesia
- Persistence of the causative infection or superinfection because of the ulceration
- Inflammation without infection, such as in the stomach
- Peptic and other secretions
- Neoplasia
  - Ulceration of a surface carcinoma
  - Ulceration of the skin or mucosa above a dermis or submucosa involved by neoplasia as a consequence of an inflammatory ulcer, as in Marjolin's ulcer, a squamous cell carcinoma arising in an osteomyelitic sinus
- Persistence of a cause other than the above, such as pressure or fat necrosis due to acute pancreatitis
- Systemic
  - Malnutrition
  - Diabetes mellitus
  - Cachexia
  - Immune deficiency

■ Rheumatoid arthritis

What is rheumatoid arthritis (RA)?

A multisystem disease of unknown aetiology that affects about 4% of the population in the UK. The cause is unknown but the result is an immune-mediated disease with inflammation of the synovium and destruction of synovial surfaces:

- All joint types (synovial, syndesmoses, synchondroses) may be affected
- Granulation tissue forms in the damaged synovium
- Cartilage is attacked
- The underlying bone develops local osteopaenia probably because of stimulation of osteoclasts by interleukins
- The joint capsule is destroyed
- A similar inflammatory process can also affect tendon sheaths
- Results in flexion deformities, radial deviation of the wrist, ulnar deviation of the fingers with subluxation of the metacarpophalangeal joints
- Eventually ankylosis of the affected joints such as the knee, elbow, hip

What are the extra-articular manifestations of RA?

These include:

- Rheumatoid nodules in about one-third of patients
  - Central coagulative necrosis
  - Macrophages around

- Palisaded fibroblasts
- Found in the skin especially over bony prominences, in the heart and lungs, occasionally in the CNS
- Rheumatoid vasculitis
  - Uncommon
  - High concentrations of IgG and IgM antibodies in affected vessel walls
  - Complement activation
  - Thrombotic occlusions
- Pericarditis, pleurisy, lymphocytic peritonitis
- Eye disease: scleritis usually, sometimes iriditis
- Amyloid deposition
- Tophi in the skin of the outer helix, periarticular tissues, larynx and heart

What agents are associated with RA and might be causative or contributory?

- Epstein–Barr virus (EBV) antigen sequences are similar to antigens in collagen and so antibodies against EBV might cross react
- Heat-shock protein can cross react with *Mycobacterium tuberculosis* and *Proteus mirabilis*
- Retroviruses are associated with a disease similar to RA in goats

■ Scars and scarring

What is a scar?

Healing by the process of repair in which there is deposition of fibrous tissue or, in the central nervous system, glial tissue.

List some complications of skin scars.

Scars are often considered trivial but they can cause:

- Severe pruritus, tenderness and pain
- Sleep disturbance, disruption of daily activities
- Physical deformity
- Compressive effects on vessels and nerves
- Psychosocial problems
  - Anxiety and depression
  - Stigmatisation
  - Post-traumatic stress reactions
  - Loss of self-esteem which is not closely correlated to the severity, size or location of scarring

In terms of the age of the patient and the site of the scar, what variables affect the scarring potential?

- Elderly people form scars that are smaller with less fibrous tissue but heal at the same rate as younger people
- Scars in intraoral tissues and conjunctiva can be invisible
- Scars are characteristically worse in adolescents and young adults
- Scars are characteristically worse in proportion to the amount of natural skin pigmentation
- Scars are worst in the deltoid and sternal regions

How do you classify scars?

- Typical scar
- Minimal scar
- Wide scar
  - Widening begins in the three weeks after operation
  - Flat, pale, asymptomatic
  - No elevation, thickening or nodularity
  - Knee and shoulder scars especially
- Atrophic scar
  - Flat and depressed, indented or inverted centre
  - Usually small
  - Common after acne and chickenpox
- Hypertrophic scar
  - Really a hyperplastic process, but the name has stuck
  - Raised but remains within the boundaries of the original lesion
  - Generally regresses spontaneously after the initial injury
  - Often red, inflamed, Itchy, sometimes painful
  - Occurs after burn injury on the trunk and extremities
- Keloid scar
  - Raised and spreads beyond the margins of the original wound
  - Infiltrates the surrounding normal skin
  - Not site specific but predominantly affects
    - Ear lobes
    - Central sternal area
    - Deltoid area

- Continues to grow over time
- Does not regress spontaneously
- Almost invariably recurs after simple excision
  - Intermediate scar
    - Scars that are difficult to categorise have been termed intermediate scars
  - Scar contracture
    - Cross joints or skin creases at right angles
    - Prone to develop shortening or contracture
    - Typically disabling and dysfunctional
    - Usually hypertrophic
    - Common after burn injury across joints

What are the predictors of abnormally severe scarring?
- Positive family history
- Amount of tissue loss
- Previous abnormal scarring in the same or other sites
- Poor response to treatment
- Scars in specific anatomical locations, as above
- Large size
- Continuing inflammation
- Severe symptoms

How are problematic scars managed?
- Non-invasive options
  - Compression therapy
    - Pressure garments with or without gel sheeting
    - Acrylic casts

- Static and dynamic splints
- Masks and clips
- Application of oils, lotions and creams
- Antihistamines
- Hydrotherapy
- Psychosocial counselling
- Masterly inactivity: wait for a year and review
- Invasive treatments
  - Surgical excision and resuture
    - Only if the surgeon thinks that more favourable conditions for wound healing can be provided than on the first occasion
  - Intralesional injections
    - Corticosteroids: complications include fat atrophy, dermal thinning, pigment changes
    - Fluorouracil, interferon gamma, bleomycin
  - Radiotherapy, laser therapy
  - Cryosurgery

▪ Screening

What are the principles of a national general screening programme?

A screening programme is the codified search for unsuspected disease in a population of apparently healthy people.

The disease should be:

- Common, or at least relatively so
- An important health problem
- One with a long premorbid latent period
- Asymptomatic or with only non-specific symptoms
- Detectable at an early stage
- Treatable
  - According to an accepted policy
  - In a cost effective way
  - At the time of detection by screening

The screening test should be:

- Sensitive
- Specific
- Non-invasive
- Audited
- Acceptable to patients
- Cost-effective
- Without significant harm to the screened patient in terms of the test and the information that the test reveals

Give three examples of targeted cancer screening.

- Screening for breast carcinoma
- Screening for ovarian cancer in patients at risk
  - With two or more first degree relatives with ovarian cancer
  - With the BRCA1 or BRCA2 gene, or both
- Colorectal carcinoma screening in at-risk families

In the case of screening for colorectal cancer, what are the problems?

- Lack of uptake
  - Advertising problems
  - Social class differences in regard to stool collections
  - National characteristics in regard to stool collections
- Sensitivity and specificity
- Methodology of testing
- Cost
- Delay in receiving results
- Patient distress when further assessment is needed

Give an example of a non-neoplastic disease that can be screened for.

Screening for abdominal aortic aneurism.

■ Sickle cell disease

What is sickle cell disease?

An abnormality of haemoglobin synthesis that results in a less soluble than normal haemoglobin with consequently reduced red cell survival (haemolytic anaemia) and polymerisation of haemoglobin with precipitation under low-oxygen tension.

What is the biochemical abnormality in HbS?

There is a single aminoacid substitution on the β-chain at position 6 of valine for the normal glutamic acid. The abnormal valine causes agglutination of the haemoglobin in its deoxygenated form to a less-soluble polymer.

How is the disease inherited?

As an autosomal co-dominant affecting chromosome 11. Homozygotes with two abnormal chromosome 11s have 90–100% HbS, heterozygotes with only one have 20–40% HbS.

What are the clinical features of sickle cell disease?

- Haemolytic anaemia, resulting in
  - Cardiovascular changes such as cardiac failure
  - Pigment gall stones
- Sickle cell crises with thrombosis and infarction
  - Abdominal and chest pain
  - Splenic infarction
  - Bone pain
  - Haematuria
  - Priapism

- Sequestration of red cells
  - Splenomegaly
  - Hepatomegaly
- Infection, such as salmonella osteomyelitis and pneumococcal sepsis

What is the blood picture in sickle cell disease?
- Normochromic film
- Sickled red cells
- Reticulocytosis
- Leucocytosis
- Features of splenic atrophy
  - Target cells
  - Acanthocytes
  - Howell–Jolly bodies
- Fragmented red cells
- Leucopaenia
- Thrombocytopaenia

■ Sinuses and fistulas

How are sinuses classified?

Sinuses can be:

- Anatomical and normal: coronary sinus, air sinuses, intracranial venous sinuses
- Pathological

What is a pathological sinus?

A blind ended tract that communicates with an epithelial surface, characteristically as a result of an inflammatory process (an epithelial surface in this context subsumes a mesothelial and endothelial surface) and usually lined by granulation tissue.

What is a fistula?

An abnormal communication between two epithelial surfaces (epithelial used as above) characteristically lined by granulation tissue.

Can a fistula be a normal structure?

By definition, no.

What is the commonest example of a fistula?

Ears pierced for earrings if one accepts that the two sides of an ear lobe constitute two epithelial surfaces. Perianal fistulas running from one aspect of the anus to another are accepted as true fistulas and can similarly be very short. Other fistulas include enteroenteric fistulas between one part of the small bowel and another, enterocolic, enterovesical, enterocutaneous and gastroenteric.

What factors determine the rate of healing of a sinus or fistula?

Local factors:

- Persistence of the causative agent
- Infection irrespective of the causative agent
- The amount of traffic through the fistula
- Foreign material
- The width of the sinus or fistula (but not the length as healing occurs from side to side)
- Local ischaemia
- Epidermidisation (epithelialisation) of the track
- Malignant change

Systemic factors:

- Nutrition
- Damage by radiotherapy
- Immunosuppression
- Diabetes mellitus
- Vitamin deficiency especially vitamin A

■ Skin cancer

What types of skin cancer are there?
- Basal cell carcinoma (BCC)
- Squamous cell carcinoma (SCC)
- Melanoma
- Kaposi's sarcoma (now considered to be a reaction to human herpes simplex virus type 8)
- Merkel cell tumour and other rare malignancies

What are the causes of skin cancer in general?
These include:
- Ultraviolet light
- Other ionising radiation such as X-rays
- Chemical carcinogens such as tars, dyes, rubber products
- Viruses such as human papilloma virus (HPV)
- Immunosuppression, related to viral infection
- Congenital abnormalities such as xeroderma pigmentosum and albinism, which can be related to one or more of the above
- Congenital syndromes like atypical naevus syndrome

What factors determine the prognosis of skin cancer?
- Tumour type (SCC, BCC, and so on as above)
- Tumour subtype (e.g. nodular, superficial spreading, acral lentiginous, lentigo maligna subtypes of melanoma)
- Grade

- Site of the tumour
  - Some tumours behave differently in different parts of the body, such as melanoma
  - Will determine to some extent whether or not the tumour can be fully excised
- Thickness and depth of invasion
- Stage of the tumour
- Whether the tumour is solitary or multiple
- Associated features such as AIDS and lymphoma

■ Skin protection

How does the skin protect against injurious agents?

- Physical barrier
  - High mechanical strength
  - Reinforced on palms, soles, fingernails and toenails by extra keratin
- Desquamation
  - Shedding of skin squames keeps bacterial growth down
- Filtration of light and ionising radiation
  - Epidermal cells have melanin granules which absorb the radiation
- Secretion
  - Sweat, which contains immunoglobulins and is acidic because of lactic acid
  - Sebum, which contains immunoglobulin and is acidic because of fatty acids
- Hair
  - Physical barrier
  - Advanced warning of possible contact injury
  - Protects against friction
- Commensals: protect against pathogens
- Immunological: Langerhans cells

■ Splenectomy

What are the indications for splenectomy?

- Trauma especially with splenic rupture
- As part of the staging and possibly typing of lymphoma
- As treatment of haemolytic diseases:
  - Hereditary spherocytosis
  - Thalassemia major
  - Some forms of immune thrombocytopaenic purpura
- As part of the treatment of thrombotic thrombocytopaenic purpura and hairy-cell leukaemia
- Symptomatic in massive splenomegaly
  - CMV
  - Myelofibrosis
  - Kala-azar (visceral leishmaniasis)
- For the treatment of hypersplenism
- Incidentally in some operations
  - Extensive gastrectomy
  - Whipple's operation
  - Adrenalectomy
  - Left upper colectomy
- Other lesions
  - Splenic cysts, congenital or from hydatid and other infections
  - Splenic vein thrombosis
  - Other primary or undiagnosed neoplasm (metastasis to the spleen from carcinoma is very rare)

What are the effects of splenectomy?

- Benefits of the primary indication above
- Red cell changes
  - Nucleated red cells
  - Inclusion bodies
    - Howell–Jolly bodies (nuclear remnants)
    - Heinz bodies (denatured haemoglobin)
    - Pappenheimer bodies (iron-containing granules)
  - Abnormal red cell forms: target cells, acanthocytes
- White cell changes
  - Transient neutrophilia
  - Permanent lymphocytosis and monocytosis
  - Overswing in infection with leucocytosis higher than in patients with a spleen
- Platelet changes
  - Thrombocytosis
  - Increased platelet adhesiveness
  - Abnormally large and distorted platelets
- Immune changes
  - Reduced plasma IgM concentration
  - Defective production of antibodies recognising carbohydrate-linked antigens
  - Increased risk of infection by capsulated organisms
    - *Streptococcus pneumoniae*
    - *Haemophilus influenzae*
    - *Neisseria meningitidis*
    - *Klebsiella pneumoniae*
  - Increased risk of contracting malaria
  - Increased risk of reactivating malaria

How is antibiotic prophylaxis managed?

- For all children aged up to 16 years
  - Lifelong prophylactic antibiotics should be offered in all cases, especially
    - In the first 2 years after splenectomy
    - When there is known to be impaired immune function
- In patients not allergic to penicillin
  - A supply of amoxycillin should be kept at home and taken on holiday
  - It should be used immediately if the patient develops pyrexia, malaise or shivering
    - The patient should seek immediate medical advice
- In patients taking erythromycin as prophylaxis
  - Pyrexia or shivering is an indication to increase the dose to a therapeutic level or change to a broader-spectrum antibiotic
    - The patient should seek immediate medical advice
- Antibiotic prophylaxis may not prevent sepsis
  - Phenoxymethylpenicillin does not cover *Haemophilus influenzae*
  - Amoxycillin does not cover *Haemophilus influenzae* reliably
  - Antibiotic resistance must be suspected if empirical treatment of sick patients is used
  - Local resistance patterns may indicate the need to use other antibiotics

■ Splenomegaly and hypersplenism

Define splenomegaly and list the causes.

An abnormal increase in splenic *size* and *weight*, irrespective of function.

The causes of massive splenomegaly include chronic myeloid leukaemia, myelofibrosis, kala-azar (visceral leishmaniasis) and some types of idiopathic thrombocytosis.

In general, the causes of splenomegaly include:

- Inflammation
  - Infections
    - *Viruses*: EBV, HIV, CMV, measles, hepatitis viruses
    - *Bacteria*: TB, treponaemes, brucella, typhoid
    - *Fungi*: histoplasma
    - *Protozoa*: malaria, toxoplasmosis, leishmania
    - *Metazoa*: hydatid disease
  - Non-infective inflammatory diseases
    - Sarcoidosis
    - Rheumatoid arthritis
    - Systemic lupus erythematosus
- Accumulation
  - Storage diseases: Gaucher's, Niemann–Pick; Hurler, Hunter
  - Amyloidosis
- Congestion
  - Thrombosis of splenic or portal veins
  - Fibrosis or cirrhosis of liver

- Budd–Chiari syndrome
- Right-sided cardiac failure
- Congenital reasons
  - Cysts in polycystic disease
  - Hereditary haemolytic anaemias
- Neoplasia
  - Leukaemia: any but especially chronic myeloid leukaemia
  - Other myeloproliferative disorders: polycythaemia vera, myelofibrosis, thrombocytosis, mastocytosis
  - Lymphoma: Hodgkin's disease, non-Hodgkin's lymphoma
- Iatrogenic
  - Antibiotics: pencillins, cephalosporins, sulfonamides
  - Others: heparin, thiazides, methyldopa, carbamazepine, phenytoin

What is hypersplenism?

An abnormal increase in splenic *function*, linked to size. All of the causes of splenomegaly above, especially congestive splenomegaly, can cause hypersplenism.

Features of hypersplenism include:

- Splenomegaly
- Inappropriate removal of red cells, white cells, platelets or combinations
- Normal marrow production of blood cellular components
- Reversal of blood abnormalities after splenectomy

■ Spread of infection

What are the principal sources of infection? Give examples.

- Human beings
  - Patients with active disease such as tuberculosis, measles, mumps, gonorrhoea
  - People with subclinical infections, such as influenza viruses
  - Carriers, such as of *Staphylococcus aureus*, *Neisseria meningitidis*
- Animals
  - Zoonoses in farm workers, veterinary surgeons, slaughterhouse staff
  - Transmission of infection from hides, bones
- Food
  - Food poisoning organisms such as *Clostridium perfringens* and *Salmonella* spp.
- Water
  - Contamination by faecal bacteria such as *Vibrio cholerae*
- Soil
  - Tetanus, fungal infections
- Air
  - Air has a resident flora of bacteria
  - Also bacteria from human beings (from the respiratory tract and desquamated skin particles) and in dust

What are the principal routes of infection?

- Inhalation by droplet spread
- Ingestion – faeco-oral transmission or ingestion of infected foods
- Contact spread from kissing, infected fomites
- Sexual intercourse causing infections of genitalia, anorectum and pharynx; systemic spread can occasionally occur
- Inoculation – catheterisation, injection, blood transfusion
- Insect-borne by biting insects
- Transplacental spread of viruses, other organisms

What is the difference between an endemic disease and an epidemic disease?

Essentially, time:

- An *endemic* disease exists continuously in a population, usually at a relatively low prevalence
- An *epidemic* disease is sporadic and tends to involve large numbers of people
- A *pandemic* is an epidemic that affects more than one continent

■ Staphylococci and streptococci

What are the main species of *Staphylococcus*?

- *Staphylococcus aureus*
- Coagulase-negative staphylococci including *Staphylococcus epidermidis* (formerly called *Staphylococcus albus*) and *Staphylococcus saprophyticus* which can occasionally cause urinary tract infection

What are the morphological and cultural characteristics of staphylococci?

- Gram-positive cocci arranged in clusters
- Golden colonies (*Staphylococcus aureus)* or white colonies (*Staphylococcus epidermidis*)
- Typed by their susceptibility to a panel of bacteriophages, bacterium specific viruses

What are the pathogenic properties of *Staphylococcus aureus?*

- Coagulase which clots plasma, resulting in the typical lesions of furuncles and abscesses
- Production of several types of exotoxin which cause vomiting and diarrhoea
- Fibrinolysin which digests fibrin
- Hyaluronidase which breaks down ground substance

How are streptococci classified?

- By the type of haemolysis on culture on a blood-agar plate:
  - Partial haemolysis (α): *Streptococcus pneumoniae*
  - Complete haemolysis (β): *Streptococcus pyogenes*
  - No haemolysis (γ): *Enterococcus* spp.
- By Lancefield group antigens, of which the important examples include:
  - Group A: *Streptococcus pyogenes*
  - Group B: None (*Streptococcus agalactiae*)
  - Group C: None (*Streptococcus equisimilis*)
  - Group D: *Enterococcus faecalis*
  - Group F: the *Streptococcus milleri* group which includes *Streptococcus milleri*, *Streptococcus mitis* and *Streptococcus sanguis*

What are the morphological and cultural characteristics of streptococci?

- Gram-positive cocci arranged in chains or pairs
- Transparent colonies with haemolysis in some cases
- Typed by API strips, a commercially available multifactorial analysis
- Virulence factors for Group A streptococci include:
  - Streptokinase which converts plasminogen to plasmin and so lyses fibrin
  - Hyaluronidase which breaks down ground substance
  - Streptolysin which causes breakdown of red cells
  - Pyrogenic toxins, which cause scarlet fever
- Lesions caused include spreading infection (cellulitis, lymphangitis) and glomerulonephritis

■ Sterilisation and disinfection

What do disinfection and sterilisation mean? How do they differ?

Disinfection is a process which kills or inactivates most micro-organisms but does not kill spores or all viruses.

Sterilisation is a process that removes all living micro-organisms including spores and viruses.

Which organisms are spore bearing?

Bacteria in the genera *Bacillus* and *Clostridium*, and some fungi.

What is the function of a bacterial spore?

To resist:

- Heat
- Dehydration
- Chemical attack
- Ionising radiation

How is disinfection achieved?

- Skin preparation
- Glutaraldehyde treatment of endoscopes

How is sterilisation achieved?

- Moist heat (steam under pressure)
  - Dressings, instruments
    - 134°C for 3 minutes or 121°C for 15 minutes
- Dry heat
  - Glassware
    - 160°C for over 2 hours

- Ethylene oxide
  - Plastics
  - Sophisticated instruments
- γ radiation
  - Plastics
  - Prostheses

■ Teratoma

Define a teratoma.
A teratoma is a true neoplasm that is composed of cells with the potential to form all three germ layers. Teratomas may be benign or malignant.

At which sites can a teratoma arise?
- The gonads: 99% of teratomas of the ovary are benign. All teratomas of the testis are malignant
- Other sites are rare and all mid-line
  - Pineal
  - Hypothalamus
  - Pituitary
  - Retropharyngeal tissues
  - Mediastinum
  - Pericardium
  - Posterior peritoneal wall
  - Retrosacral region

Can a benign teratoma develop malignancy?
Malignancy may rarely arise in a benign teratoma:
- Squamous cell carcinoma
- Adenocarcinoma
- Carcinoid

Testicular neoplasms I: classification and germ cell tumours

How are testicular neoplasms classified?

Primarily into germ cell neoplasms and non-germ cell neoplasms.

How are germ cell tumours classified?

Testicular germ cells normally make or contribute to:

- More germ cells as in seminoma
- Fetal tissues, and hence mature adult tissues; teratomas are defined as being composed of cells that have the potential to differentiate into cells from all three germ lines: ectoderm, mesoderm and endoderm
- Placental tissues

The classification of germ cell neoplasms reflects this:

- Seminoma
  - Classical type
    - Typical seminoma
    - Anaplastic seminoma
  - Spermatocytic seminoma
- Teratoma
  - Teratoma differentiated
    - Classified as teratoma by the World Health Organization (WHO)
    - With or without malignant elements such as squamous cell carcinoma of the skin or

adenocarcinoma of the bowel in a testicular teratoma

- Malignant teratoma intermediate
  - Classified as embryonal carcinoma with teratoma by WHO
  - Commonest type
  - Composed partly of mature tissues and partly of undifferentiated tissues
  - The more the undifferentiated tissue element, the worse the prognosis within this group
- Malignant teratoma undifferentiated
  - Classified as embryonal carcinoma by WHO
  - No differentiation (or very little differentiation) into mature tissues
- Malignant teratoma trophoblastic
  - Placental development
  - Classified as choriocarcinoma by WHO
  - Rare in the pure form
  - Poor prognosis
- Yolk sac tumour (sometimes called endodermal sinus tumour but human beings do not have endodermal sinuses)
  - Placental (or related) development
  - Usually occurs as a part of a mixed germ cell tumour
  - Associated with a favourable prognosis as the relapse rate after treatment is statistically lower

Testicular neoplasms II: prognostic indicators

What are the prognostic indicators for a patient with testicular germ cell neoplasm?

- The tumour type: patients with
  - Seminoma have a very good prognosis
  - Spermatocytic seminoma have an even better prognosis
  - Mature teratoma have a very good prognosis though metastasis is still possible
  - Pure yolk sac tumours (usually in infants) have a very good prognosis
  - Undifferentiated and trophoblastic tumours have a poor prognosis though it is improving with advances in chemotherapy
  - A neoplasm other than a germ cell tumour
- The histopathological features of the tumour: indicators of a poor prognosis include
  - Blood vessel invasion
  - Lymphatic invasion
  - Presence of undifferentiated teratoma
  - Absence of yolk sac elements
- The tumour stage
  - Stage 1: tumour confined to the testis
  - Stage 2: involvement of lymph nodes (LNs) below the diaphragm, classically para-aortic nodes

- Stage 3: involvement of LNs above and below the diaphragm
- Stage 4: extranodal metastases

What is the prognosis of the rare tumours of the testis that are not germ cell tumours?

Germ cells normally are associated with sex cord cells, Sertoli cells, and the stromally derived cells of the testis, Leydig cells. Neoplasia of these cells can occur separately or together. Leydig cell tumours are the commonest of this rare group:

- Leydig cell tumours
  - About 2% of testicular neoplasms
  - Form a testicular mass
  - Are associated with gynaecomastia as they can secrete testosterone and oestrogens
  - Are associated with precocious puberty in boys
  - Can histologically resemble testicular nodules of ectopic adrenal cortex in the testis when they are stimulated by congenital adrenal hyperplasia
  - Behave in a malignant fashion in 10% of cases when the tumour arises in an adult; in children the natural history is benign
- Sertoli cell tumours
  - Rare testicular neoplasms
  - Associated with gynaecomastia, especially when the Sertoli cell tumour is malignant
  - More aggressive in patient older than 10 years

■ Tetanus

What is tetanus?

Tetanus is a disease of the CNS caused by tetanospasmin ascending up the motor nerve trunks and interfering with the inhibitory processes of motor neurones. There is therefore increased muscle tone related to the area of infection in the first instance but spreading to involve other areas.

What are the characteristic clinical signs of tetanus?

Tetanospasmin is transported from the site of infection to the CNS where it binds to presynaptic inhibitory motor nerve endings and inhibits the release of inhibitory neurotransmitters. This results in:

- Trismus from masseter spasm ("lock jaw")
- Spasm of facial muscles ("risus sardonicus")
- Dysphagia
- Opisthotonus
- Tetanic convulsions
- Death from asphyxia

How is tetanus prevented?

- Immunisation with tetanus toxoid, a denatured preparation of the toxin, to stimulate immunity
  - Long lasting
  - Does not prevent infection with *Clostridium tetani*, only prevents the toxin acting

- Treatment with human antitetanus immunoglobulin if a high risk patient is not immune because of previous toxoid immunisation
  - Short duration
  - May cause anaphylaxis
  - Prevents infection with *Clostridium tetani* temporarily

■ Thalassaemia

What is the intrinsic defect in thalassaemia?
Defective globin chain synthesis causing abnormal haemoglobin production and disordered erythropoiesis.

How is thalassaemia classified?
- α-thalassaemia affects patients especially in China, elsewhere is Asia, Africa
- β-thalassaemia affects patients especially in Mediterranean countries, Middle East

What is the blood picture in a patient with thalassaemia?
- Hypochromic, microcytic anaemia
- Reticulocytosis
- Target cells
- Nucleated red cells
- Increased fetal haemoglobin on electrophoresis

What are the complications of thalassaemia?
- Marrow hyperplasia
- Iron overload
  - Cirrhosis
  - Endocrine disturbances
  - Pancreatitis
- Hypersplenism
  - Decreased red cell survival time
  - Leucopaenia
  - Thrombocytopaenia

■ Thrombocytopaenia

What does thrombocytopaenia mean, and how does it differ from thrombasthenia?

- Thrombocytopaenia is a reduction below normal of the number of platelets
- Thrombasthenia is a reduction below normal of the function of platelets irrespective of number. Some conditions cause both

Classify the causes of thrombocytopaenia.

- Failure of production
  - Aplastic anaemia
    - Congenital: Fanconi's anaemia
    - Drug-induced: cytotoxic drugs, drugs causing hypersensitivity states
    - Radiotherapy and accidental radiation exposure
    - Autoimmune causes with no known aetiology
    - Others: viral infections, pregnancy
  - Megaloblastic anaemia
  - Myelodysplastic syndromes other than idiopathic thrombocythaemia
  - Bone marrow replacement by metastatic carcinoma
  - HIV and other virus infections
  - Congenital causes (rarely)
    - May–Heglin anomaly
    - Bernard–Soulier syndrome
    - Osteopetrosis with obliteration of the marrow

- Increased platelet consumption
  - Disseminated intravascular coagulopathy
  - Immunological causes
    - Antibodies against drugs
    - In a blood transfusion reaction (post-transfusion purpura)
    - Idiopathic thrombocytopaenic purpura
    - Heparin-induced thrombocytopaenia
    - Diseases such as systemic lupus erythematosus (SLE) and anti-phospholipid syndrome
  - Malaria, glandular fever, schistosomiasis
  - Thrombotic thrombocytopaenic purpura
  - Splenomegaly and hypersplenism (sequestration mostly with little degradation)
- Relative thrombocytopaenia
  - Dilutional
    - Large transfusions of fluid such as dextrose saline
    - Large blood transfusion with stored blood low in platelets
  - Artefactual thrombocytopaenia
    - Some patients have antibodies that cause aggregation of platelets in glass tubes, and so appear to have thrombocytopaenia

Classify the causes of thrombasthenia.

- Congenital
  - Platelet membrane glycoprotein abnormalities
    - Glanzmann's thrombasthenia: autosomal recessive disorder

- Bernard–Soulier disease: autosomal recessive disorder, large platelets
  - Storage granule abnormalities
    - Storage pool disease: deficiency of dense granules, alpha granules, or both resulting in defective release of ADP and serotonin
- Acquired
  - Drugs
    - Aspirin inhibits prostaglandin synthetase and prevents release of ADP and thromboxane A2
    - Furosemide, sympathetic blockers, clofibrate, non-steroidal anti-inflammatory drugs, nitrofurantoin, heparin
  - Chronic renal disease with uraemia
  - Chronic liver disease with jaundice

■ Thrombosis and clotting

How is a clot different from a thrombus?

A clot is solid material formed from the constituents of blood in *stationary* blood. Clotting is essentially a function of the intrinsic or extrinsic clotting cascade.

A thrombus is solid material formed from the constituents of blood in *flowing* blood. Thrombosis is essentially a function of platelets, and only secondarily a function of the clotting cascade.

In the context of a thrombus what are the functions of platelets?

- Adhesion to a vessel wall which, in the presence of von Willebrand factor (factor VIII complex) leads to shape change and degranulation
- Aggregation with contraction to form a dense solid mass in a vessel
- Release of compounds such as prostaglandins, serotonin and thromboxanes that have effects on vessels walls and other tissue cells

What factors contribute to thrombosis?

Virchow's triad: changes in the vessel wall, the blood constituents and the blood flow.

What changes in the vessel wall contribute to thrombosis?

- Atheroma

- Direct trauma from heat, cold, mechanical damage, chemical injury
- Iatrogenic from cannulation, radiotherapy

What changes in the blood constituents contribute to thrombosis?

- Thrombocytosis
- Increase in coagulation factors, such as fibrinogen
- Coagulant compounds released from malignancies
- Hyperviscosity from hypergammaglobulinaemia, polycythaemia
- Inherited deficiencies of protein C, protein S and antithrombin III (natural anticoagulants)
- Iatrogenic: injection of sclerosants for the treatment of varicose veins, embolisation of renal cell carcinoma

What changes in the flow of blood contribute to thrombosis?

- Atheroma changing the speed and flow though arteries
- Reduction in flow in patients who have compromised venous drainage, such as in the deep veins of the leg
- Local stasis in aneurysms
- Turbulence from artificial valves, stents, implanted devices

■ Thyroid cancer: thyroid neoplasms

What are the main five thyroid neoplasms seen in general surgical practice?

Papillary, follicular, medullary and anaplastic carcinoma, and thyroid lymphoma.

Why are the carcinomas classically ordered in that way?

The order relates to prevalence and prognosis.

What are the characteristics of a papillary carcinoma?

- Has a prevalence of about 80% of thyroid carcinomas
- Is multifocal in as many as half of cases
- Is diagnosed incidentally in apparently normal glands in 2–5% of post-mortem examinations
- Classically metastasises via lymphatics to local LNs: small palpable tumours are associated with LN metastases in 50% of cases, large tumours in 80% of cases
- Is related to exposure of the thyroid to radiation, either therapeutically or after escape of radiation from nuclear power plants
- Has a histological appearance that is distinctive irrespective of the behaviour of the neoplasm in terms of its invasiveness
- Has a prognosis of about 90% after 5 years

What are the characteristics of a follicular carcinoma?

- Has a prevalence of about 15% of thyroid carcinomas
- Is rarely multifocal, is rare as an incidental finding at post-mortem and is unrelated to radiation exposure
- Classically metastasises relatively early through the bloodstream to bone marrow and lungs; LN metastases are unusual
- Has a histological appearance that is usually bland. Diagnosis does not depend on the appearance of the tumour cells themselves but on their behaviour. It is necessary to demonstrate capsular invasion or invasion of vessels at the periphery of the tumour
- Has a prognosis of about 70% after 5 years

What are the characteristics of a medullary carcinoma?

- Has a prevalence of 5–8% of thyroid carcinomas
- Is associated with multiple endocrine adenopathy (MEA) II syndromes. Spontaneous medullary carcinoma (70%) is usually unilateral: genetically determined medullary carcinoma (30%) is almost always bilateral
- Is derived from thyroid C cells which make calcitonin. This stains with Congo red with apple-green dichroic birefringence and so is amyloid. The histological appearance is distinctive
- Metastasises to LN and bone marrow
- Has a prognosis of about 90% after 5 years, if at excision it is confined completely within the thyroid, 70% if local LNs have metastases, and 20% if other tissues are involved. Overall it has a 5-year survival of about 60%

What are the characteristics of an anaplastic carcinoma?

- Has a prevalence of 2–5% of thyroid carcinomas
- Arises in iodine-deficient areas or on a background of existing thyroid disease such as multinodular goitre or a differentiated carcinoma
- Metastasises early to local and distant sites through lymphatic and blood vessels
- Has a distinctive histological appearance with sheets of highly mitotic and atypical cells
- Has a 5-year prognosis of zero. 10% of patients survive for 3 years

Can thyroid cancer be diagnosed on fine needle aspiration (FNA)?

All except one:

- All papillary neoplasms are malignant: there is no entity of papillary adenoma
  - Almost all of them can be diagnosed on FNA
  - Depends on the finding of tumour papillae
- No follicular lesion can be given a definite diagnosis on FNA
  - The differential includes a follicular adenoma, follicular carcinoma, dominant nodule in a multinodular gland, colloid nodule and an enlarged intrathyroid parathyroid gland (which also may have follicles)
  - The diagnosis depends on the *histological* demonstration of invasion of the capsule or peripheral vessels
- Medullary carcinoma is usually easy to diagnose, with regular boxy cells in an amyloid matrix that can be seen on the cytology preparation

- Anaplastic carcinoma is easy to diagnose; the anaplasia is usually very obvious

What type of lymphomas affect the thyroid?

- Non-Hodgkin's lymphoma (NHL) in almost all cases: primary Hodgkin's disease of the thyroid is very rare
- NHL is associated with Hashimoto's disease and occasionally with Graves' disease
- NHL of the thyroid has two main variants, the aggressive and the indolent types. Most are aggressive and numerous lymphocyte types are involved
- Thyroid NHL accounts for 3% of all cases of NHL: 5% of all thyroid cancers are NHL
- The indolent variant is associated with mucosa-associated lymphoid tissue (MALT)
- FNA diagnosis is possible but may be difficult as it can resemble anaplastic carcinoma and lymphocytic throiditis
- Surgery is not indicated: chemotherapy has good effects without excision
- The prognosis is about 85% at 5 years

Thyroid overactivity: excess thyroxine or T3

What are the causes of hyperthyroidism?

- Graves' disease
- One or more hyperactive nodule in a multinodular goitre
- Follicular adenoma
- Early Hashimoto's disease
- Carcinoma of the thyroid
- Overtreatment with thyroxine
  - Replacement after thyroidectomy
  - Treatment of hypothyroidism
- Other drug-induced causes
  - Amiodarone therapy
  - Radiological investigations using iodine-based contrast
  - Medium
- Pregnancy

Rare causes:

- Basophil adenoma of pituitary
- Struma ovarii: thyroid tissue in a dermoid cyst of ovary

What do the terms *hot* and *cold nodule* refer to?

Uptake on a radioactive iodine scan:

- Hot: 95% benign and 5% malignant
- Cold: 80% benign and 20% malignant

How are T4 and T3 synthesised?

Iodination of tyrosine results in mono-iodotyrosine and di-iodotyrosine. Coupling of these results in tri-iodothyronine and tetra-iodothyronine (Note the different suffix: tyrosine has one benzene ring and thyronine has two).

■ TNM staging

What are the principles of the TNM method of staging neoplasms?

The system was developed in the 1950s for:

- Management
- Indication of prognosis (in combination with many other factors)
- Evaluation of the results of treatment
- Formalisation of minimal data sets for histological reporting and in clinical trials

The aim was that there should be no ambiguity and few value judgements. The system is based on the anatomical extent of the tumour only.

- What do T, N & M stand for?
  - T is the size & local extent of the tumour
  - N is the presence of *regional* LN metastasis
  - M is the presence of distant metastasis *including* LN metastasis

In brief, what are the components of the TNM system for staging?

These comprise:

- The categories of local involvement by the tumour
  - TX: the primary tumour cannot be assessed
  - T0: no evidence of the primary tumour (such as after radiotherapy)
  - Tis: carcinoma in situ
  - T1–T4: size and local extent of the tumour

- The categories of LN involvement
  - NX: regional nodes cannot be assessed
  - N0: no regional node metastases
  - N1–N3: extent of regional node involvement
- The categories of distant metastases (including distant LN metastases)
  - MX: distant metastases cannot be assessed
  - M0: no distant metastases
  - M1: distant metastases are present (their site is stated here)

A potentially confusing addition is that there are C categories (called C1–C5) based on evidence from clinical information including imaging and R categories (called RX–R2) to indicate the extent of residual disease after treatment. These should not be confused with the cytological assessment and radiological assessment of breast cancer (called C1–C5 and R1–R5) in which the categories are entirely different.

▣ Treponemal diseases

Classify the treponemal diseases

- Venereal
  - Syphilis: *Treponema pallidum* ssp. *pallidum*
- Non-venereal
  - Yaws: *Treponema pallidum* ssp. *pertenue*
  - Bejel: *Treponema pallidum* ssp. *endemicum*
  - Pinta: *Treponema carateum*

An awareness of endemic, non-venereal forms of treponemal infection is important because of misinterpretation of serological tests that suggests syphilis.

What are the characteristics of a treponeme?

Treponemes belong to the family Spirochaetacea. They are motile, spiral organisms that flex in the middle as they move (a spirillum is similar but does not flex).

Of the treponemal diseases, which are endemic and which are sporadic?

Syphilis is sporadic, the rest are endemic.

Where are they endemic?

North and Middle Africa, Central and South America, Middle East, Indonesia, Borneo, Papua New Guinea.

Why are treponemal diseases of surgical importance?

In the differential diagnosis of:

- Orthopaedic abnormalities
- Cardiothoracic abnormalities

- Paediatric facial abnormalities
- Neurosurgical abnormalities such as space-occupying lesions in the brain

What other organisms are included in the genus of spirochaete?

- *Borrelia* spp.
  - In the human mouth as commensals
  - In animals, passed to man by ticks and lice such as Lyme disease
- Leptospira found in animals, ditches and streams

■ Tuberculosis

What organism is tuberculosis caused by?
- *Mycobacterium tuberculosis* var. *hominis* in man
- *Mycobacterium tuberculosis* var. *bovis* in cows

How is tuberculosis classified clinically?
- Primary tuberculosis which is usually symptomless in the UK
- Post-primary tuberculosis in which there is cough, fever, weight loss. Limited spread of infection by a severe local response with cavitation and fibrosis

What are the typical sites of involvement for primary tuberculosis?
- Lung, by far the commonest
- Tonsils, with cervical LN involvement (scrofula)
- Terminal ileum, with mesenteric LN involvement ("tabes mesenterica" – the term is now obsolete)

What is the primary complex in an affected lung?
The association of the local lesion (Ghon focus) with involvement of lymphatics and enlargement of hilar LNs. The Ghon focus characteristically forms at the periphery of the lung in the mid-zone on a chest X-ray.

How may the primary lesion in tuberculosis progress to cause more generalised disease?

- Haematogenous spread leading to
    - Miliary tuberculosis in many organs
    - Tuberculous meningitis
    - Bone and joint tuberculosis
    - Renal tuberculosis
    - Tuberculous epididymitis
- Spread by rupture into air spaces leading to
    - Tuberculous bronchopneumonia

What is the characteristic site of involvement in post-primary tuberculosis?

The lungs, either by reactivation of latent organisms or reinfection. An Assman lesion forms, usually at an apex, and often cavitates and heals by dense fibrosis with consequent emphysema to form a lung cavity.

◼ Tumour markers

What is a tumour marker?

A substance reliably found in the circulation of a patient with neoplasia which is directly related to the presence of the neoplasm, disappears when the neoplasm is treated and reappears when the neoplasm recurs.

No tumour marker is pathognomonic, but many aid diagnosis and most are used for surveillance.

Tumour markers are not usually stoichiometric – the amount produced is not in direct proportion to the tumour bulk – but carcinoembryonic antigen (CEA) has been shown to be reliably so.

How are tumour markers classified in terms of their biochemical structure or function?

As hormones, isoenzymes and oncofetal and other protein antigens.

How may hormones be used as tumour markers?

Hormones may be produced by tumours eutopically or ectopically.

If there is a neoplasm of the pituitary or adrenal gland, for example, there may be production of ACTH, hGH, PRL or another pituitary hormone, or of cortisol or aldosterone.

Ectopic hormone production occurs with carcinoid tumours and other neuroendocrine neoplasms.

Give examples of isoenzymes as tumour markers.

- Prostatic acid phosphatase for carcinoma of the prostate
- Placental alkaline phosphatase for neoplasms of germ cells and carcinoma of the bronchus, pancreas and colon

Give examples of oncofetal antigens.

- α-fetoprotein for germ cell tumours, hepatocellular carcinoma
- CEA for colorectal carcinoma (limited use, as levels rise in several different types of carcinoma and in inflammatory conditions)

What tumour markers are characteristically found in testicular tumours?

- Teratoma: β-hCG, CEA, α-fetoprotein
- Seminoma
  - Placental alkaline phosphatase
  - β-hCG if the seminoma has multinucleate giant cells

Are proliferation markers the same as tumour markers?

Proliferation markers are non-specific and unreliably related to the presence of neoplasms. They include:

- Ploidy measurements on flow cytology which measure the mean DNA content (irrespective of chromosome number or size)
- S-phase markers on flow cytometry which measure the proportion of tumour cells that are in the synthesis phase of the cell cycle

- Receptors and growth factors
  - Oestrogen receptor (ER), progesterone receptor (PR) and HER 2
  - Insulin-like growth factor
  - CD44 and heat-shock proteins, measures of metastatic potential and invasiveness
  - p53 gene product

■ Ultraviolet light

How does ultraviolet (UV) light and other ionising radiation cause damage to cells?

- Direct DNA damage
  - TT dimer formation: abnormal links between thymidine bases instead of the normal AT links
  - Base deletions
- Indirect damage to DNA by free radicals (usually minor as UV is not very high energy but important in xeroderma pigmentosum)

What tissues are especially at risk of damage by UV light (especially in sunlight)?

- The skin: especially skin types 1 and 2, and in people with types 3–6 at the junction of the sole and the pigmented skin of the foot
- The cornea

What are the pathological changes in the skin caused by UV light?

- Inflammation of the skin
- Wrinkles, scarring, abnormal pigmentation
- Solar elastosis
- Neoplasia
  - Basal cell carcinoma
  - Squamous cell carcinoma
  - Melanoma

How are tissues classified in terms of their capacity to regenerate after damage?

- *Labile cells and tissues*: bone marrow, testis, small and large bowel
- *Stable cells and tissues*: liver, kidney, adrenal, bone
- *Permanent cells and tissues*: CNS, skeletal muscle

Is this directly commensurate with their capacity to resist the damaging effects of radiation?

No.

■ Urinary tract calculi

What are urinary tract calculi characteristically composed of?

- Oxalate and mixed oxalate: phosphate stones
  - Account for about three-quarters of all urinary tract calculi
  - Spiky or mulberry shapes
  - Caused by hypercalciuria usually
  - Hyperoxaluria is rare, caused by
    - An inherited enzyme deficiency
    - Coeliac disease, diverticula of the small bowel and chronic pancreatitis in which oxalate absorption from the diet is increased
- Magnesium ammonium phosphate
  - Account for about one-sixth of all urinary tract calculi
  - Associated with Proteus infection
- Urate
  - Account for about one in twenty of all urinary tract calculi
  - Primary gout
    - Hypoxanthine guanine phosphoribosyl transferase deficiency
    - Decreased fractional excretion of urate
  - Secondary gout
    - Increased purine (not pyrimidine) breakdown in
      - Spontaneous necrosis in malignant tumours

- ▲ Treatment by radiotherapy or chemotherapy of malignancies such as myeloproliferative disorders
- ▲ Severe psoriasis
- Cysteine
  - Account for about 3% of all urinary tract calculi
  - Usually the result of primary cysteinuria, an inborn error of metabolism
- Xanthine

What are the complications of urinary calculi?

- Obstruction by the calculus itself, if in the ureter or possibly urethra
- Obstruction as a consequence of fibrosis from irritation and ulceration by the calculus
- Hydroureter and hydronephrosis
- Ascending infection
- Squamous metaplasia and rarely squamous cell carcinoma
- Iron-deficiency anaemia from chronic blood loss (rare)

◼ Urinary tract infections

What constitutes a urinary tract infection (UTI)?
Infection of the bladder, the ureters and the kidney via the renal pelvis. Infection of the urethra is not usually considered to be a UTI but rather a sexually transmitted disease (STD).

Which patients are predisposed to contracting UTIs?
- Women, because of
  - The proximity of the urethra to the anus in a moist environment
  - Honeymoon cystitis
  - Length of the urethra (questionable)
- Patients who have been catheterised
- Causes of urinary stasis
  - Prostatic enlargement
  - Cystocele
  - Neurogenic bladder
  - Bladder calculus causing fibrosis
  - Schistosomal infection
  - Hydronephrosis
- Congenital abnormalities affecting urine flow
  - Ectopia vesicae
  - Duplication of ureter
  - Urethral valves or congenital stricture
  - Incompetence of the vesico-ureteric junction with reflux
- Patients with diabetes, immune deficiencies

What organisms characteristically cause UTIs?

- *Escherichia coli*
    - Especially strains that have capsular antigens that inhibit phagocytosis and the bactericidal effects of complement
- *Proteus mirabilis*
- *Pseudomonas aeruginosa*
- *Klebsiella* spp.
- *Enterococcus* spp. (new term for *Streptococcus faecalis*)
- *Staphylococcus aureus*

How is a UTI diagnosed?

- Microscopy for white cells and organisms
- Culture of a midstream specimen of urine
- Fewer than 10^3 organisms/ml is not considered to be significant. More than 10^5 organisms/ml in pure culture is empirically considered to be an infection
- A midstream urine sample minimises contamination from meatal or urethral commensals. An early morning urine (EMU) specimen with a midstream catch is suitable (an EMU should not be used for cytological examination for malignant cells – any epithelial cells present will be degenerate and difficult to interpret)

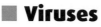 Viruses

How are viruses classified?

Principally by the type of nucleic acid and the shape:

- Type of nucleic acid: DNA virus or RNA virus
- Size and shape: parvovirus, picornavirus, rhabdovirus, small round virus

Also by:

- Diseases that they cause: measles, mumps, yellow fever, poliomyelitis
- The types of tissue that they infect: adenoviruses infect glands, enteroviruses infect the bowel
- Effects on tissues: human papilloma virus (HPV), herpes virus (herpes means creeping)

Name some important DNA viruses.

- Herpes virus causing mouth and genital ulceration, chicken pox and shingles; general infections in patients with AIDS; infectious mononucleosis and possibly Burkitt's lymphoma and nasopharyngeal carcinoma
- HPV causing squamous cell papilloma and carcinoma
- Hepatitis B virus causing hepatitis and cirrhosis
- Pox virus causing molluscum contagiosum and orf
- Adenovirus causing infections of the upper and lower respiratory tract, the small bowel and bladder, and the eye

Name some important RNA viruses.

- Influenza virus
- Human immunodeficiency virus (HIV)

- Rubella virus
- Togavirus causing rubella. Intrauterine infection can lead to severe abnormalities in the ears, eyes, heart, lungs and liver
- Coronavirus causing the common cold and severe acute respiratory syndrome (SARS)
- Orthomyxovirus and paramyxovirus causing influenza and parainfluenza
- Rhabdovirus causing rabies in canines, rodents and bats
- All of the hepatitis viruses except for Hepatitis B

■ Viruses and neoplasia

How are viruses related to neoplasia?
- Viruses can directly cause neoplasia
- Viruses can cause diseases that predispose to neoplasia
- Neoplasms provide a new substrate for viruses and so neoplasms can become infected by viruses without them being in any way causative

What viruses cause neoplasia?
Viruses that have been associated causally with neoplasia include:
- HTLV1 and adult leukaemia of T-cell type
- Epstein-Barr virus (EBV) and Burkitt's lymphoma
- EBV and nasopharyngeal carcinoma
- HPV and cervical, skin, perineal and anal carcinoma

What viral diseases predispose to neoplasia?
- Hepatitis B virus infection causing chronic active hepatitis progressing to cirrhosis and possibly hepatocellular carcinoma. Hepatitis D (which is an incomplete virus, called a virusoid) is a co-factor especially in South East Asia
- HIV causes an immunodeficiency state which is permissive for HPV and for the development of lymphomas

■ Wounds I: wound infection

How are wounds classified in terms of the problems with bacterial and other contaminants?

Into the four classical types of wound:

- Clean wound
  - Alimentary tract not breached
  - Respiratory tract not breached
  - No inflammation evident
  - No fault in aseptic technique
- Clean contaminated wound
  - Alimentary tract breached but without significant spillage
  - Respiratory tract breached
  - No inflammation evident
  - No fault in aseptic technique
- Contaminated wound
  - Significant spillage from a hollow organ such as bowel
  - Active inflammation with pus formation
  - Significant fault in aseptic technique
  - Fresh traumatic wounds
- Dirty wound
  - Obvious pus formation
  - Old traumatic wound

How are the factors that predispose to wound infection classified?

Factors that relate to the

- Patient
  - Local ischaemia
  - Metabolic factors: jaundice, diabetes mellitus, uraemia, inadequate nutrition or obesity
- Infecting organism
  - Virulence
  - Dose
  - Antimicrobial resistance
- Wound
  - The type of wound relative to its cause: clean, contused, lacerated, avulsed, puncture
  - Drainage of the site: spontaneous, surgically-aided

What is sepsis?

The development of a systemic inflammatory response syndrome (SIRS) as a result of infection.

SIRS is characterised by two or more of the following:

- Temperature above 38.4°C or below 35.6°C
- Pulse rate above 90 beats/minute
- Respiratory rate above 20 breaths/minute or $PaCO_2$ less than 32 mmHg
- White cell count
  - More than 12,000 cells/ml
  - Less than 4,000 cells/ml
  - More than 10% band forms (neutrophil precursors)

Wounds II: causative injury and haemostasis

How are wounds classified in terms of the damage caused by the causative injury?

Into open and closed wounds:

- Open wounds
  - Clean: surgical incision, knife wounds without complications, broken clean glassware
  - Contused: an element of crushing contributing to the wound
  - Lacerated: an element of stretching, tearing or explosion
  - Avulsed: degloving injury to a digit or penis with full-thickness skin displacement
  - Superficial puncture: splinters, thorns, spicules of glass, nails
  - Deep puncture: impalement, stabbing
  - Missile
    - Superficial or deep
    - Single or multiple
    - Low or high velocity
- Closed wounds
  - Contusions without skin breach: crush, bruising
  - Haematoma formation
  - Fracture: bone, penis

What are the principles for achieving haemostasis?

Avoidance of the causes of blood loss and control of blood loss if this is not possible.

- Avoidance of blood loss
  - Ligature or clip; double ligature or suture ligature on large vessels
  - Tourniquet
  - Adrenaline instillation
  - Cutting diathermy
  - Cutting laser
- Control of blood loss
  - Direct pressure and heat; packs, compression bandages
  - Ligation or clipping
  - Gell-foam, powdered collagen preparations
  - Coagulating diathermy
  - Coagulating laser

How are surgical dressings classified?

By their function or functions:

- As a pressure bandage
- As a temporary seal
- As protection against
  - Infection
  - Abrasion
  - Inadvertent damage by the patient such as an infant or child
  - Dehydration
- Absorbence: of pus, blood, exudate

An on-line index is available at http://www.dglowe.com